FAT ACTIVISM

FAT ACTIVISM

A RADICAL SOCIAL MOVEMENT

Charlotte Cooper

HammerOn Press

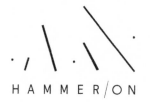

HAMMER/ON

Charlotte Cooper's fierce new book *Fat Activism: A Radical Social Movement* should be required reading for scholars and activists. Cooper draws on extensive interviews with fat activists to render a trenchant analysis of our field of motion. She takes a penetrating look at activist efforts and self-understandings, eschewing easy praise in favour of discernment that ultimately promises to invigorate the movement.

Kathleen LeBesco / Marymount Manhattan College (Associate Dean)

For any civil rights movement to succeed, it must know its history; to build on its strengths and learn from its mistakes. With the ubiquity of the Internet, the historical knowledge and record of activism can be rewritten with 140 characters. That is one of the many reasons that *Fat Activism: A Radical Social Movement* is important. Charlotte's latest text provides a detailed presentation of fat activism throughout the twentieth and twenty first centuries, including illumination of those who have appropriated and occupied fat activism for their own agendas. She highlights the achievements of fat activism, while also acknowledging where it has often failed (for example, the dominance of the work in the United States, the often limited accessibility, the lack of intersectionality). Charlotte allows space for both assimilationist and anti-assimilationist activism, closing the text with delightful examples of her own work as a queer fat activist. Anyone interested in the epistemology, ontology, and methodology, (not to mention history) of fat activism should make this a central text of their library.

Cat Pausé / Massey University / Co-Editor of *Queering Fat Embodiment*

Charlotte Cooper is once again in the vanguard of radical social change with this book about fat activism. She has captured the history of the fat rights movements, interviewed fat activists, and demonstrated the extensive and exciting breadth of fat activism in a global setting. Fat activism is often portrayed as ineffective when in fact its lack of conformity and interdisciplinarity can serve as a model for other social movements.

Esther Rothblum / Editor / *Fat Studies: An Interdisciplinary Journal of Body Weight and Society*

It is in the interest of the ethically and intellectually dubious field of "Obesity Research" to flatten fat subjects; rendering our voices narrowly defined by punchy rhetoric, our activist interventions reduced to child-like flailing against the big bad thin-dominated world. Charlotte Cooper's book *Fat Activism: A Radical Social Movement* resists this myopic view of resistance to fat oppression in form and content. By remaining true to her own subject position as a Fat Activist who works in community with other Fat Activists, Cooper lays out a methodology and practice of fat studies research that positions lived experience at the center of her rigorous analysis. This book is full of honesty about the challenges of doing research on a complex, diverse community, and acknowledges its own pitfalls and under-developed critiques gracefully. Fat Activists need more researchers and writers examining and reflecting on our work from within, and this book stands as an offering and opening in that vein.

Naima Lowe / Artist and Member of the Faculty at The Evergreen State College

FAT ACTIVISM: A RADICAL SOCIAL MOVEMENT
© Charlotte Cooper, 2016

The right of Charlotte Cooper to be identified as Author of
this work has been asserted in accordance with the Copyright,
Designs and Patent Act 1988

ISBN-13: 978-1-910849-00-2
ISBN-10: 1910849002

Fat Activism: A Radical Social Movement/ Charlotte Cooper
1. Social Movement Studies 2. Fat Studies 3. Public Health
4. Obesity 5. Cultural Studies 6. Feminism 7. Lesbian, Gay,
Bisexual, Transgender, Queer.

First published in 2016 by HammerOn Press
Bristol, England
http://hammeronpress.net

Cover design by Eva Megias
http://evamegias.com

ACKNOWLEDGMENTS

It has taken me years to write this book. I am grateful to everybody who consented to be interviewed for this project, all the reviewers and every single one of the hundreds of people who offered me words of encouragement and opportunities to share this work. Thanks to Simon Murphy, Kay Hyatt, Deborah Withers, Eva Megias, Natalie Brown, Ann Kaloski Naylor, The Institute for the Study of Knowledge in Society, The Irish Social Sciences Platform and Sociology at Limerick.

CONTENTS

For you.

INTRODUCTION

Fat[1] people are a fact of life, part of the fabric of humanity. There is evidence that we have existed for many thousands of years.[2] We are here. There are many who would prefer fat people not to exist, but we are here regardless of whether or not we are allowed or supposed to be here. Fat people are as valuable as anyone else and our existence reveals

1   I consider fat a form of non-normative embodiment relating to the presence of adipose tissue. I resist using Body Mass Index to measure or categorise fat because I reject the medicalisation, moral stratification, and commercial exploitation of fat bodies that BMI engenders. Similarly, I am unable to name a weight at which one becomes fat because this disregards the diversity of how people embody fatness, or are socially positioned as fat. Like all bodies, fat bodies are not static, they age, they get fatter and thinner over time, they may become increasingly or less disabled, they may be changed by disease, decoration, or the life course, and they are socially constructed. There is no universal measure or mark that constitutes what is and what is not fat; fat exists in context and experience; fat people know who they are and are known as fat by others. The use of the word fat is controversial and has been criticised as strident and alienating. Bovey, Shelley. *Sizeable Reflections: Big Women Living Full Lives* (London: Women's Press, 2000). I prioritise fat over medicalised language (obese, overweight, bariatric), euphemisms (large, big, weight, curvy), terms of endearment (cuddly, big-boned), or other interpretations (of size, thick) because I wish to acknowledge it as a descriptive word, a reclaimed word that contests shame, a political word that expresses power and exposes the limitations of those other linguistic constructions.
2   The Venus of Willendorf is the oldest figure of a human subject in existence, a fat black woman between 25 and 28 thousand years old. Shaw, Andrea Elizabeth. *The Embodiment of Disobedience: Fat Black Women's Unruly Political Bodies* (Lanham, MD: Lexington Books, 2006). Megalithic fat figures in Malta are much younger, only 2500-4000 years old. Still, both massively pre-date present day fat panic also known as the obesity epidemic.

important things about how societies operate. As a psychotherapist, I am interested in the ways in which people might grow towards hopes and dreams, express agency, by which I mean the capacity to choose and act independently, even within restrictive social contexts; to really live. I see activism as a strategy for developing what Judith Butler calls "liveable lives" in contexts that are extremely trying, as well as creating social change.[3] How can and do fat people try to make liveable lives for ourselves and others? That's basically what this book is about.

I begin by examining what others have already said about fat activism[4] which, in my opinion, is quite limited and does not reflect my own decades-long experiences of the movement or its everydayness. I go on to argue that different kinds of research methods are needed in order to unlock knowledge that has already been generated by fat people. I describe how my peers do fat activism and I locate these actions in historical and geographical contexts. I ask "How did fat activism reach me?" and chart a particular genealogy from coastal USA in the late 1960s to Europe in the 1980s and beyond. I show that fat activism has enjoyed an expansiveness that is currently being stalled by conservative values and I end by encouraging fat activists to resist the pull of access and assimilation, if they can, and consider queer[5] strategies to reinvigorate the movement.

I am writing in a context where being fat is commonly experienced in the West[6] at this moment in time as being at best pretty awful. But this is

3 Judith Butler, *Undoing Gender* (New York: Routledge, 2004).
4 In this study I use the terms fat activism, fat liberation, fat politics, fat pride, fat rights, the movement somewhat interchangeably to describe a social movement concerned with fatness that has many sites and interests. Other people use fat acceptance and size acceptance.
5 I will write about queer in more depth later but for now I will define this indefinable term as both a means of talking about sexuality and a quality, a sensibility of not fitting in and unsettling oddness.
6 There are many definitions of the West and throughout this book I use it to refer to liberal democratic capitalist regions, cultures and values influenced by ancient Greece and Rome, as well as Christianity, and which are allied with or settler products of Western Europe and North America.

not a book about obesity, a word I use to describe the idea that fatness is a problem in need of a solution, or the obesity epidemic, a rhetorical device to leverage fat panic.[7] Although there is plenty that is awful about how fat people are treated, that awfulness is not at the heart of this book either. I think of shame as political, not a natural inevitability. I am not going to explore whether or not fat people are healthy, the prime concern in the world of obesity, although I am very much interested in how fat people cope with being treated as unhealthy.[8] Neither will I explore whether or not fat people are a drain on resources, a factor in global warming, a symptom of over-consumption or a product of obesogenic environments.[9] People preoccupied with how fat people can be caused, managed and prevented will not find much about it here.

The dominance of anti-obesity rhetoric means that dissent is usually understood as being part of a debate. In this book I present fat activism as a social movement, not a debate. That is to say, it is a concept that is not always concerned about participating in this debate or in need of validation through it, it exists regardless of whether or not there is a debate, and it has done for some years. When I say social movement I mean the actions that people take that often have some connection to social change

7   Michael Gard and Jan Wright, *The Obesity Epidemic: Science, Morality, and Ideology* (Abingdon: Routledge, 2005); Michael Gard, *The End of the Obesity Epidemic* (Abingdon: Routledge, 2011); Natalie Boero, *Killer Fat* (New Brunswick, NJ: Rutgers University Press, 2012). Most accounts of fat panic are orientated towards the US, but Friedrich Schorb makes a good stab of historicising its development in Europe. Friedrich Schorb, "Fat Politics in Europe: Theorizing on the Premises and Outcomes of European Anti-'Obesity-Epidemic' Policies," *Fat Studies: An Interdisciplinary Journal of Body Weight and Society* 2, no. 1 (2013): 3-16.

8   The shouts of fat feminists from 35 years ago echo: "THE SUPPRESSION OF INFORMATION ABOUT FAT PEOPLE'S HEALTH AND NUTRITION IS A MAJOR POLITICAL PROBLEM". Judith A Stein and Beryl-Elise Hoffstein, *Proceedings of the First Feminist Fat Activists' Working Meeting: April 18-20, 1980, New Haven, Ct.* (Minneapolis, MN: Fat Liberator Publications, 1980).

9   Rachel Colls, Bethan Evans and Elaine Graham-Leigh do a much better job of that than I. Rachel Colls and Bethan Evans, "Making Space for Fat Bodies? A Critical Account of 'the Obesogenic Environment,'" *Progress in Human Geography* 1, no. 21 (2013); Elaine Graham-Leigh, *A Diet of Austerity: Class, Food and Climate Change* (London: Zero Books, 2015).

and which are bound together by various threads to do with history, place, philosophy, identity and so on, of which this book is full of examples. Fat activism is an idea that connects many different kinds of people and activities and contributes to how people think of social action, social change and social movements. Fat activism shows that you do not have to be corralled into a debate in order to think, speak and act.

Fat Activism: A Radical Social Movement is linked to another book, *Fat & Proud: The Politics of Size*, not least because they are both based on my academic work and desire to see ideas move beyond the world of the university. In that other book I developed a theory, suggested to me by my friend and mentor Jenny Corbett, that the Social Model of Disability could be applied to fat activism.[10] This means that instead of trying to normalise fat people through dodgy medical interventions, or demonising our bodies, it would be better if society was able to accommodate us. This book maintains that basic assumption but is a product of more sophisticated and rigorous research, it asks bigger questions of fat activism and is more critical of the movement. This book is the first time that such a broad and in-depth ethnography[11] of fat activists by a fat activist-researcher has taken place. Like my previous book, this one is based on primary evidence and has a moderately international scope. It is also a book that is openly queer, something that the publishers of *Fat & Proud* tried to suppress.

The book you are reading started out as my doctoral research at the University of Limerick in Ireland, which began in 2008 and ended

---

10   Others have since built on this work. Hannele Harjunen, "Exploring Obesity through the Social Model of Disability" in *Gender and Disability Research in the Nordic Countries*, edited by Traustadóttir Rannveig and Kristjana Kristiansen, 305-24 (Lund: Studentlitteratur, 2004); Lucy Aphramor, "Disability and the Anti-Obesity Offensive," *Disability & Society* 24, no. 7 (2009): 897-909; Nathan Kai-Cheong Chan and Allison C. Gillick, "Fatness as a Disability: Questions of Personal and Group Identity," *Disability & Society*, no. 2 (2009): 231-43; Toby Brandon and Gary Pritchard, "'Being Fat': A Conceptual Analysis Using Three Models of Disability," *Disability & Society*, 26, no. 1 (2011): 79-82.

11   An ethnography is a study of people that tries to convey their point of view or what it is like to be them.

in 2012. The study was originally proposed by my supervisors to the funding body as a piece of research about anti-fat discrimination in the dietetic clinic. It would add to an evidence base of anti-fat bias and stigma, and an emerging literature of critical dietetics.[12] The proposal reflected my supervisors' and the funders' interests more than mine and did not consider the possible effect on a fat researcher, such as I, of encountering relentless clinical discrimination over at least a four-year period. A different approach was required that reflected my experience and knowledge of fat, which built on my expertise as a fat activist, enabled me to write myself into the research, and which posed less of a risk to my well-being. The original proposal made a brief mention of resistance to clinical discrimination. Fat activism was regarded as a minor footnote even here! A short course on peace-building undertaken at the end of my first year of study, which included a module on community strategies for non-violence, convinced me that activism needed to be central to the study.

This change of focus transformed the work. Instead of research that reproduced fat people's helplessness and marginalisation, which dwelt on fat hatred and abjection, or reinforced medical supremacy, or the power of the expert, or reiterated claims about anti-fat discrimination that are already well-worn and deeply known to fat people, I was free to explore the political imaginations of fat community. I could say something new.

12 Jeffrey M Friedman, "A War on Obesity, Not the Obese," *Science* 299, no. 5608 (2003): 856-59; Mary Madeline Rogge and Marti Greenwald, "Obesity, Stigma, and Civilized Oppression," *Advances in Nursing Science* 27, no. 4 (2004): 301-15; Sondra Solovay, "Remedies for Weight-Based Discrimination," in *Weight Bias: Nature, Consequences and Remedies*, edited by K. D Brownell et al, 212-22 (New York: The Guilford Press, 2005); Lucy Wang, "Weight Discrimination: One Size Fits All Remedy?" *Yale Law Journal* 117, no. 8 (2008): 1900-45; Linda Bacon and Lucy Aphramor, "Weight Science: Evaluating the Evidence for a Paradigm Shift," *Nutrition Journal*, 10, no. 9 (2011): na; Amy Erdman Farrell, *Fat Shame: Stigma and the Fat Body in American Culture* (New York: New York University Press, 2011); Stephanie von Liebenstein, "Confronting Weight Discrimination in Germany – the Foundation of a Fat Acceptance Organization," *Fat Studies: An Interdisciplinary Journal of Body Weight and Society* 1, no. 2 (2012): 166-79; Amanda Marie Balkhi, Mike C. Parent and Mark Mayor, "Impact of Perceived Weight Discrimination on Patient Satisfaction and Physician Trust," *Fat Studies: An Interdisciplinary Journal of Body Weight and Society*, 2, no. 1 (2013): 45-55.

The work would not be governed by obesity, stigma, normativity,[13] or
health, the usual ways by which fat is framed, but could reflect other ways
of knowing. The research focused on fat people rather than professionals,
on actions that take place in multiple contexts rather than in the clinic, on
a wide range of social activity rather than that limited to health or food.
Because I am a part of fat community as well as a researcher, it became
a piece of work by and of a group of people, and for them. It was and is
one of the rare occasions in which agentic fat people are positioned at
the centre of the work as narrators.

Fat Activism: A Radical Social Movement is the product of an emerging
interdisciplinary field called Fat Studies. Fat Studies puts fat in the middle of
an academic and research discourse, there is no need to justify its presence.[14]
Fat people are active and visible as contributors to Fat Studies. It could be
argued that Fat Studies represents a type of activism in itself because it
acknowledges the political nature of the work. Two key anthologies map the
field as it stands, but continue a trajectory of earlier critical analysis in the
work of Hillel Schwartz and in collections edited by Jana Evans Braziel and
Kathleen LeBesco.[15] In the UK, a series of Economic and Social Research
Council seminars helped establish Fat Studies between 2010-2011 and
I was proud to deliver the keynote at the first one. Fat Studies conferences
have taken place in the United States, Australia and New Zealand, and 2012
marked the publication of the first issue of Fat Studies: An Interdisciplinary
Journal of Body Weight and Society.[16]

13 Normative or normativity is a way of saying standard, socially constructed as
normal, idealised, morally correct. What is normal changes in different contexts.
14 When I use the word discourse, which I do a lot in this book, I mean "all the things
in that particular realm or universe." So obesity discourse means "all the associations
that spring to mind when fat people are thought of as being a disease in need of a cure."
15 Hillel Schwartz, Never Satisfied: A Cultural History of Diets, Fantasies and Fat (New
York: The Free Press, 1986); Jana Evans Braziel and Kathleen LeBesco, Bodies out of
Bounds: Fatness and Transgression (Berkeley: University of California Press, 2001);
Corinna Tomrley and Ann Kaloski Naylor, Fat Studies in the Uk (York: Raw Nerve
Books, 2009); Esther Rothblum and Sondra Solovay, The Fat Studies Reader (New York:
New York University Press, 2009).
16 Esther D. Rothblum, "Why a Journal on Fat Studies?" Fat Studies: An Interdisciplinary
Journal of Body Weight and Society 1, no. 1 (2012): 3-5.

I hope that *Fat Activism: A Radical Social Movement* enjoys a broad readership, I see it as a book for anyone interested in the subject. But as I have been writing, there are particular people that I have kept in mind as groups to whom I am trying to speak directly.

The first, of course, are fat activists. This book could not exist without my own experience as a fat activist, which permeates the work. I see myself as a cultural worker, a term that I think came out of a communist aesthetic of the early 20th century.[17] I see culture-making as political, as *work,* not something magical that is mysteriously conjured by special people. I am grateful to Elana Dykewomon for introducing me to this concept in relation to fat lesbian feminism. In an oral history recorded in Oakland, she mentions that cultural workers are invested in community rather than celebrity or stardom.[18]

The second group are researchers. One of the reasons that obesity research is in crisis is because of its endemic marginalisation, dehumanisation and exploitation of fat people. This book represents a different way of knowing and finding out about fat. It reflects a conviction that obesity research must address fat activism if it is to be ethical, and that fat activism should consider adopting the values of Research Justice if it is to transform knowledge. I draw on knowledge produced beyond the usual academic databases which underpins so much work in the field and is, to my mind, quite tired. Instead this book reflects the vitality of embodied community knowledge, it is grounded in a long-term struggle for social change. Conversations and home-made objects are my data, and I draw predominantly on fat feminist perspectives developed by

---

17   John Pietaro, "The Cultural Worker," http://theculturalworker.blogspot. co.uk/2010/12/communist-cultural-workers-brief.html.

18   "A cultural worker is somebody who is part of a community and the art that they make it comes from their experience in that community and is a part of the dreams and aspirations and critical understanding of that community". Andrew Leland, "Elana Dykewomon: An Oral History," Oakland Museum of Calfornia, http://museumca.org/theoaklandstandard/elana-dykewomon-oral-history. See also Elana Dykewomon, "Changing the World" in *Everyday Mutinies: Funding Lesbian Activism,* edited by Gartrell Nanette and Esther D. Rothblum, 53-62 (Binghampton: Harrington Park Press, 2001).

the commons, not through high level obesity policy. This is critical in enabling communities to appreciate their power. I have decided not to conform to academic orthodoxy to speak only to a research community through journal articles hidden behind expensive pay walls, or costly monographs written in arcane language. Although this study reflects scholarly conventions to some extent, I speak and write with a voice that I hope is accessible to many and I avoid or explain jargon where possible. It is a para-academic project in this respect and also because I am no longer firmly attached to a pedagogical institution.[19] This book is not a tool to help me get a good job or become a professor. I am lucky to be working with a publisher supporting this perspective, I encourage other researchers to use similar tactics and seize opportunities to do research about fat activism both in and beyond institutions.

The agents of obesity discourse and public health promotion are the third group towards whom this work is directed. This is unavoidable in the current climate. Anti-obesity strategies currently involve speculative and costly investment in disrupting energy balance,[20] food taxation and marketing, coercive physical activity, genetic engineering, pharmacological and surgical interventions and sanctions against fat people, as well as public-private partnerships with the weight loss industry.[21] Yet fat activists have already developed sustainable low cost

19   Jamie Allen, "Discussions before an Encounter," *continent* 2, no. 2 (2012): 136-47; Alex Wardrop and Deborah M. Withers, eds. *The Para-Academic Handbook: A Toolkit for Making-Learning-Creating-Acting* (Bristol: HammerOn Press, 2014).

20   The dominant rationale for fat in obesity discourse, energy balance refers to an equation where body weight is the result of a relationship between energy consumed, through eating food, and energy expended, through physical activity. Where more energy is consumed than expended, overweight and obesity results. This is a contested model but it remains common sense knowledge.

21   Glen Gaesser, *Big Fat Lies: The Truth About Your Weight and Your Health* (Carlsbad, CA: Gurze Books, 2002); Paul F. Campos et al, "The Epidemiology of Overweight and Obesity: Public Health Crisis or Moral Panic?" *International Journal of Epidemiology* 35, no. 1 (2006): 55-60. Susan Stinson explains why economic sanctions against fat people further marginalise those on the edges and ignore the problem of the corporate greed of weight loss industries Susan Stinson, "Nothing Succeeds Like Excess: Corporate Greed Goes Unchecked in a Fat-Phobic Society," *The Women's Review of Books* XVIII, no. 10-11 (2001): 16.

and low risk strategies for living well that are adaptable to different circumstances. What would obesity research and policy look like if the interventions and approaches that I describe in this book were taken seriously? The beneficial impact of appropriate and sensitive services or policies on the well-being of humankind is beyond current imagination. But this would require that fat activists become recognisable by institutions where invitations to act as their consultants can be double-edged. Challenging systemic fatphobia[22] requires systemic social change, this is likely to be beyond the scope of the organisation, or to contradict its interests. Institutions are not necessarily the places where queer fat feminist activism, or that which is weird or unconventional, can flourish. By becoming institutionalised or adopted as policy, actions might no longer be called activism. Appropriation is a possibility, and the likelihood of egalitarian anti-oppressive collaboration between policy-making institutions with interests in obesity and fat activists remains doubtful right now.[23] Meanwhile, though present, obesity policymakers are background figures in this work for the simple reason that fat activists do not need their permission, influence or money to act.

As a research project this book is a snapshot of a period of about four years, as a depiction of fat activism it reflects my social networks of that period and my own histories. These are always contextual and in process, there's no end point. I invite readers to treat me – and all researchers – as an unreliable narrator of fat activism. Although I will argue that I am in a better position to write about the movement than many others who have already tried, and that who gets to speak about fat activism or represent it is very important and highly political, my account is also limited because of who I am. I have tried to include lots of different voices and perspectives in this book, but I am one person and cannot speak for all, nor would I want to. So I wish to state the obvious:

22 The fear and hatred of fat people.
23 See, for example, the mess that the anti-fat Obesity Action Coalition has made in trying to introduce patronising people first language and anti-stigma projects whilst upholding an oppressive disease model of fat. Obesity Action Coalition. "Obesity Action Coalition." www.obesityaction.org/.

Fat Activism: A Radical Social Movement is not the first or the last word about fat activism, it is not definitive. Readers should keep in mind that this book is about how *I* see things, it is not a complete account, as if such a thing could exist. There is room for more than one book about fat activism and one of my hopes for this work is that it encourages others to speak, share, publish and disseminate their own knowledge.[24]

There should be many books and conversations about fat activism. To do this means creating access, making platforms, making space, it cannot be the work of tenured academics. It must ensure that grassroots voices are always cherished and supported, as I have tried to do here.

Charlotte Cooper
London, 2016

charlottecooper.net

24 I encourage activists to learn how to cite each others' work, to recognise what we do as work, gifts or contributions. This helps create a trail for other activists and researchers and it contests the belief that academia is the only place where important ideas emerge.

UNDOING

This chapter begins with me undoing a series of assumptions about fat activism and inviting readers to question what they know about the movement. One of the motivations for writing this book was my dissatisfaction with the majority of popular and scholarly writing about fat activism. I am interested in and dismayed by the ways that official, allegedly rigorous knowledge gets cited, reproduced, sanctioned and treated as definitive whilst distorting or disengaging with what fat activists actually do. I see this happening all the time within obesity discourse and it happens in critical accounts too. Sometimes I think that the only allowable fat person in research is one who is absent, silent and complicit.

I have called these assumptions proxies. They emerge from accounts of fat activism that have been most cited, although they rarely reflect my experiences as a fat activist. A proxy is a stand-in, or someone authorised to represent someone or something else. Proxies are jargon, a partial view, shorthand, a grain of something small that ends up becoming absolute. With these proxies, particular facets of fat activism are taken to represent the movement as a whole and, as a result, problematic assumptions arise.

Later on, I will explain that these proxies predominate because research into fat, and especially fat activism, is currently very limited and this affects the kinds of knowledge about it that exists. Towards the end of the chapter I describe how I went about researching fat activism for this book. I talk about the theories that made sense to me and the methods I used. Using different methodologies to research fat activism creates different ways of knowing about the subject, knowledge that is hopefully more relevant to fat activists.

PROXIES

I offer two sets of proxies here, they appeared again and again in my reading around fat activism. Firstly, those where fat activism is present, for example within the idea of body positivity, or the belief that NAAFA[1] is all that fat activism can be. Secondly, those in which fat activism is obscured by other concerns, including body image, the obesity epidemic, health and stigma.

FAT ACTIVISM IS ABOUT BODY POSITIVITY

This proxy has its basis in Marilyn Wann's landmark publication *Fat!So? Because you don't have to apologise for your size!* which, at the moment, is most often cited by people writing about fat activism.[2] This brightly coloured activity book is written with an upbeat can-do tone and invites its readers to disinvest in self-hatred and weight loss and develop critical approaches to those concepts. Contrasting with earlier books[3] Wann makes fat activism a compelling and amusing proposition through peppy language, personal anecdotes, craft activities and quizzes presented with a cut and paste pop art visual style. The work echoes through texts by other charismatic fat activists, often successful bloggers, who have followed in Wann's footsteps to become celebrities of the movement.[4] Body positivity,

---

1 National Association to Advance Fat Acceptance NAAFA. "Naafa Online." http://www.naafaonline.com/. I will say more about this organisation later in the book.
2 Marilyn Wann, *Fat!So? Because You Don't Have to Apologize for Your Size!* (Berkeley CA: Ten Speed Press, 1998).
3 See, for example, the more sober style of Lisa Schoenfielder and Barb Wieser, *Shadow on a Tightrope: Writings by Women on Fat Oppression* (San Francisco: Aunt Lute, 1983).
4 Wendy Shanker, *The Fat Girl's Guide to Life* (New York: Bloomsbury, 2005); Lara

self-acceptance and self-love are presented as fundaments of fat activism in these works, and are achieved through self-help regimes, the work of personal growth and development, self-knowledge and reflection, the enjoyment and appreciation of other fat people.[5] The style is cheerful and evangelical and has been applied to countless fat activist interventions.

There have been minor turns within this literature. Fatshion[6] influenced earlier works.[7] More recently this has resurfaced through a plethora of blogging and related publishing, which alludes to the transformative power of access to stylish clothes.[8] Sometimes attention was more explicitly on health and fitness.[9] Later texts diversified into sexual and

Frater, *Fat Chicks Rule! How to Survive in a Thin-Centric World* (New York: Ig Publishing, 2005); Kate Harding and Marianne Kirby, *Lessons from the Fat-O-Sphere: Quit Dieting and Declare a Truce with Your Body* (New York: Perigee, 2009); Golda Poretsky, *Stop Dieting Now: 25 Reasons to Stop, 25 Ways to Heal* (Astoria, NY: Body Love Wellness, 2010); Lesley Kinzel, *Two Whole Cakes: How to Stop Dieting and Learn to Love Your Body* (New York: The Feminist Press, 2012); Ragen Chastain, *Fat: The Owner's Manual: Navigating a Thin-Obsessed World with Your Health, Happiness, and Self-Esteem Intact* (Austin, TX: Sized for Success Multimedia, LLC, 2012); Brittany Gibbons, *Fat Girl Walking: Sex, Food, Love, and Being Comfortable in Your Skin...Every Inch of It* (New York: Dey Street Books/HarperCollins, 2015); Jes Baker, *Things No One Will Tell Fat Girls: A Handbook for Unapologetic Living* (Berkeley, CA: Seal Press, 2015); Bevin Branlandingham, "The Queer Fat Femme Guide to Life," http://queerfatfemme.com/.

5 Nancy Barron, "I Like the Me I'm Becoming" in *Journeys to Self-Acceptance: Fat Women Speak*, edited by Carol Wiley, 112-23 (Freedom, CA: The Crossing Press, 1994); Bernadette Lynn Bosky, "Some Painful and Healing Words" in *Journeys to Self-Acceptance: Fat Women Speak*, edited by Carol Wiley, 54-64 (Freedom, CA: The Crossing Press, 1994); Kim Brittingham, *Read My Hips: How I Learned to Love My Body, Ditch Dieting and Live Large* (New York: Random House, 2011).

6 A portmanteau of fat and fashion, originally a fat activist critique of fashion.

7 Nancy Roberts, *Breaking All the Rules: Looking Good and Feeling Great No Matter What Your Size* (London: Penguin, 1987); Suzan Nanfeldt, *The Plus-Size Guide to Looking Great* (New York: Plume, 1996).

8 Kira Cochrane, "Young, Fat and Fabulous," *The Guardian*, http://www.guardian.co.uk/theguardian/2010/jan/30/fat-fashion-blogs; Kate Dailey, "'Fatshion' Blogs Defiantly Celebrate Plus-Size Couture," *BBC*, http://www.bbc.co.uk/news/magazine-16259070.

9 Pat Lyons and Debby Burgard, *Great Shape: The First Fitness Guide for Large Women* (Authors Guild Backinprint.com ed. Palo Alto, CA: Bull Publishing Company, 1990); Steven Jonas, *Just the Weigh You Are: How to Be Fit and Healthy, Whatever Your Size* (New York: Houghton Mifflin, 1997).

reproductive health.[10] There are also a number of celebrity memoirs that draw upon a fat activist proxy of self-love.[11] With some exceptions[12] these texts reproduce a universalised US, urban, usually white and mainly middle class culture that treats fat activism as the products of exceptional individuals now gifted to ordinary readers. As these are popular works, there is negligible theorising and analysis of the movement as a whole.

With its emphasis on 'positivity,' body positive fat activism looks very similar, in my opinion, to the positive psychology movement.[13] Critics of that movement contend that it is banal or superficial; that it promotes the idea that failure is predicated on not having tried hard enough to succeed; that there is an aggressive and coercive element to the philosophy; and that systemic inequality is overlooked particularly when the tools and methods of positive psychology have been used to further marginalise people who are struggling.[14]

Samantha Murray's criticisms of body positive fat activism fit with these broader criticisms of positivity, although she too mistakenly regards it as a proxy for the movement as a whole.[15] She is one of a

10 Hanne Blank, *Big Big Love: A Sourcebook on Sex for People of Size* (Emeryville, CA: The Greenery Press, 2000); Cornelia van der Ziel and Jacqueline Tourville, *Big, Beautiful, and Pregnant: Expert Advice and Comforting Wisdom for the Expecting Plus-Size Woman* (New York: Marlowe & Co, 2002).

11 Mo'Nique, and Sherri A. McGee, *Skinny Women Are Evil: Notes of a Big Girl in a Small-Minded World* (New York: Atria Books, 2004); Dawn French, *Dear Fatty* (London: Century, 2008); Beth Ditto and Michelle Tea, *Coal to Diamonds* (London: Simon & Schuster, 2012).

12 Virgie Tovar, ed. *Hot & Heavy: Fierce Fat Girls on Life, Love and Fashion* (Berkeley, CA: Seal Press, 2012); Sonya Renee Taylor, "The Body Is Not an Apology," http://thebodyisnotanapology.com/.

13 Martin Seligman, *Learned Optimism: How to Change Your Mind and Your Life* (New York: Knopf, 1991).

14 Barbara Ehrenreich, *Smile or Die: How Positive Thinking Fooled America and the World* (London: Granta, 2010); Lynne Friedli and Robert Stearn, "Positive Affect as Coercive Strategy: Conditionality, Activation and the Role of Psychology in UK Government Workfare Programmes," *Medical Humanities* 41, no. 1 (2015): 40-47.

15 Samantha Murray, *The 'Fat' Female Body* (Basingstoke: Palgrave Macmillan, 2008). Foucault and Butler acknowledge that self-authorship is problematic, yet they also accept that people have agency. Michel Foucault, "Power and Strategies" in *Power/Knowledge: Selected Interviews and Other Writings, 1972-1977*, edited by Michel Foucault and Colin

group of people, including Shelly Bovey, Kira Cochrane, Ann Cahill and Susanne Brandheim who have at times identified with fat activism or feminist analyses of fat but maintain an ambivalent relationship with it.[16] These authors criticise body positivity because, like many others, they feel that they cannot live up to an apparently monolithic ideal of trite self-love that mirrors diet culture with its fantasies of transformation and happy endings. They cannot conform to an activist orthodoxy of self-acceptance when their lived experience is saturated with ambivalence and pain. They want an end to their suffering as fat women and have not found it in fat activism. Instead they feel failed by a movement that they characterise as naïve, self-satisfied and out of touch with the reality of self-hatred, a movement that's as bad as or worse than a culture in which weight loss is valued. Bovey and Murray have pursued weight loss since first encountering fat activism, Bovey through a commercial dieting group and Murray via a gastric band. Their disdain for the proxy has led to work that should be of great interest to fat activists. Both authors maintain critical accounts of what weight loss entails, including its maintenance, and the management of other people's reactions.[17]

Gordon, 134-45 (Brighton: The Harvester Press, 1980); Judith Butler, *Undoing Gender* and Judith Butler, *Precarious Life: The Powers of Mourning and Violence* (London: Verso, 2004).

16 Shelley Bovey, *Being Fat Is Not a Sin* (London: Pandora, 1989); Shelley Bovey, *What Have You Got to Lose? The Great Weight Debate and How to Diet Successfully* (London: The Women's Press, 2001); Samantha Murray, "(Un/Be)Coming Out? Rethinking Fat Politics," *Social Semiotics* 15, no. 2 (2005): 153-63; Kira Cochrane, "The Reluctant Dieter," *The Guardian*, http://www.theguardian.com/lifeandstyle/series/thereluctantdieter; Ann J. Cahill, "Getting to My Fighting Weight," *Hypatia* 25, no. 2 (2010): 485-92; Charlotte Cooper and Samantha Murray, "Fat Activist Community: A Conversation Piece," *Somatechnics* 2, no. 1 (2012): 127-38; Susanne Brandheim, "The Misrecognition Mind-Set: A Trap in the Transformative Responsibility of Critical Weight Studies," *Distinktion: Scandinavian Journal of Social Theory* 13, no. 1 (2012): 93-108.

17 Bovey, *What Have You Got to Lose? The Great Weight Debate and How to Diet Successfully*; Nikki Sullivan and Samantha Murray, *Somatechnics: Queering the Technologisation of Bodies* (Farnham: Ashgate Publishing Ltd., 2009); Samantha Murray, "Women under/in Control? Embodying Eating after Gastric Banding," *Radical Psychology* 8, no. 1 (2009).

Bovey no longer identifies with fat activism but Murray maintains an on-going relationship with it, to some extent.[18]

Lily Rygh Glen has written about her feelings of exclusion from body positive fat activism because of having had an eating disorder.[19] Her claims have more substance than the other critics here, for example *Fat & Proud* is consciously distanced from earlier feminist approaches to eating disorders because of how that work had stereotyped fat people.[20] LeBesco also notes that the idea that fat people are not responsible for their weight is a politically strategic position but one which re-pathologises those whose eating habits contribute to their fatness, including people who have eating disorders.[21] Indeed, Rygh Glen's article was attacked when it was published, adding to her case that the relationship between fat activism and feminist eating disorder discourse is fraught, although more recently fat activists have been playing with some of this imagery.[22]

The criticisms offered by these authors suggest that fat activism as a project of body love is not representative of the whole. But they also have major limitations. Shelley Bovey and Murray base their claims about fat activism on sporadic disappointing encounters with this particular proxy and are unequipped to speak about fat activism with more complexity. Their difficulty in finding helpful strategies or developing supportive

18 Cooper and Murray, "Fat Activist Community: A Conversation Piece."

19 Lily Rygh Glen, "Big Trouble: Are Eating Disorders the Lavender Menace of the Fat Acceptance Movement?" *Bitch Magazine: Feminist Response to Pop Culture*, no. 38 (2008): 40-45.

20 Susie Orbach, *Fat Is a Feminist Issue: How to Lose Weight Permanently – without Dieting* (London: Arrow Books, 1978); Aldebaran (Vivian Mayer) "Letter: Compulsive Eating Myth," *Off Our Backs* 9, no. 7 (1979): 28; Marion Woodman, *The Owl Was a Baker's Daughter: Obesity, Anorexia Nervosa and the Repressed* (Toronto: Inner City Books, 1982); Kim Chernin, *The Hungry Self: Women, Eating and Identity* (New York: Times Books, 1985); Charlotte Cooper, *Fat & Proud: The Politics of Size* (London: The Women's Press, 1998).

21 Kathleen LeBesco, *Revolting Bodies: The Struggle to Redefine Fat Identity* (Amherst, MA: University of Massachusetts Press, 2004).

22 Marty Fink, "It Gets Fatter: Graphic Fatness and Resilient Eating in Mariko and Jillian Tamaki's Skim," *Fat Studies: An Interdisciplinary Journal of Body Weight and Society* 2, no. 2 (2013): 132-46.

alliances within body positive fat activism is taken as evidence of its universal lack of substance or validity, rather than a problem with one aspect of the movement. In their books neither Bovey nor Murray describes sustained involvement in collective activity, there is scarce examination of community, they are alone as fat women, without evidence of wider political or cultural engagement that might help make sense of fat activism. Rygh Glen's critique is similarly too narrow, she does not take into account work that combines fat activism and feminist eating disorder discourse, for example in Allyson Mitchell's art.[23] The fat activism they encounter is not an instant fix for their problems and it is false to assume that it can deliver answers on the same terms as the unfulfilled promises made through weight loss rhetoric.[24]

Meanwhile, Kelli Dunham's work is also of interest here because it deepens the critique of this proxy into intersectional[25] fat activism. Instead of reiterating the fundament of loving one's body, she draws on trans narratives of embodied ambivalence to develop strategies for medical self-advocacy. Dunham argues that you do not have to love your body in order to try and take care of it.[26] She demonstrates that self-acceptance or body positivity do not have to be at the core of embodied activism, including fat activism.

---

23 Allyson Mitchell, "Pissed Off," in *Fat: The Anthropology of an Obsession*, edited by Don Kulick and Anne Meneley, 211-25 (London: Penguin, 2005).

24 Jeanne Courtney, "Size Acceptance as a Grief Process: Observations from Psychotherapy with Lesbian Feminists," *Journal of Lesbian Studies*, 12, no. 4 (2008): 347-63.

25 Intersectionality means thinking about the ways that different oppressions intersect on people's identities. It is an idea founded in black feminism. Kimberlé Crenshaw, "Demarginalizing the Intersection of Race and Sex: A Black Feminist Critique of Antidiscrimination Doctrine, Feminist Theory and Antiracist Politics," *University of Chicago Legal Forum* (1989): 139-67; Linda Bean et al, "Body Consciousness," *Spare Rib* 182 (1987): 20-21; Barbara Burford, "The Landscapes Painted on the inside of My Skin," *Spare Rib*, no. 179: 36-39.

26 Kelli Dunham, "I Promise You Can Successfully Get a Pap Exam Even If You Are Traumatized, Grossed out or Really Really Not into Those Parts," xojane, http://www.xojane.com/healthy/i-promise-you-can-get-a-pap-exam-even-if-you-are-traumatized-weirded-out-grossed-out-or-really-really-not-into-those-bits.

FAT ACTIVISM IS NAAFA

This proxy operates through the belief that fat activism is a North American affair, sometimes exported elsewhere, that takes place through organisations, the only one of which worth citing being NAAFA. But fat activism is a movement and not an organisation, it happens through different places and spaces and I will show that organisations are often least engaged with by activists. Some fat activists are extremely critical of NAAFA and many do not know what it is.[27]

NAAFA is intelligible as activism because, in its public face at least, it undertakes a standard form of political process activism that is generally familiar in the West as activism, about which I will say more shortly. Thus the concepts of organisations, hierarchy, leadership and universal agendas are reproduced as the only legitimate style of fat activism in the world.[28] For example:

> [Marilyn] Wann is the current Activism Chair on the Board of Directors at NAAFA and her book is akin to a manifesto for the fat rights movement.[29]

This is not to deny Wann's influence, but the authors' hyperbole is substantiated. NAAFA as a comprehensive proxy for fat activism has been further represented as a meat market, politically conservative, and consisting of a membership of ambivalently fat people who are struggling to make sense of themselves.[30] These reductive claims do not stand up.

I suspect that this proxy has arisen, particularly in scholarly literature,

27 Kate Harding, "Dear Naafa," http://kateharding.net/2007/06/24/dear-naafa/.

28 Abigail C. Saguy and Kevin W. Riley, "Weighing Both Sides: Morality, Mortality, and Framing Contests over Obesity," *Journal of Health Politics, Policy & Law* 30, no. 5 (2005): 869-921.

29 Samantha Kwan, "Framing the Fat Body: Contested Meanings between Government, Activists, and Industry," *Sociological Inquiry,* 79, no. 1 (2009): 25-50.

30 Debra L. Gimlin, *Body Work: Beauty and Self-Image in American Culture* (Berkeley: University of California Press, 2002).

because NAAFA, and organisations where fat people come together, are important sites for researchers, especially those normatively-sized scholars who have limited contact with the movement.[31] Marcia Millman's much-cited study of NAAFA established this practice.[32] Her scholarship was ground-breaking for its time because it showed that fat people with a critical grasp of their fatness, usually women, are rich ethnographic objects, and that fat activist spaces make compelling sites for researchers.

The proxy of fat activism being NAAFA or an organisational space that is revealed by researchers raises questions about privilege and exploitation. Authors' motivations, power and positioning in relation to the movement are either not explicit, or treated as a minor detail. Richard Klein's smug encounters with members of the *FaT GiRL* collective drip with his own unexamined power in relation to gender and class.[33] Other ethnographies are more mindful of the relationships between the researcher and the researched.[34] Thin privilege flourishes through career-making studies of fat people which enable academics to climb the ranks whilst reproducing fat people as fascinating but passive specimens and enshrining knowledge within elitist educational institutions. Sometimes scholarly remove undermines the quality of the research.[35] Fat people are often spoken for by expert-professionals and denied a public voice. Sometimes these works are exploitative. As a researcher Millman

31 Paul F. Campos, *The Obesity Myth: Why America's Obsession with Weight Is Hazardous to Your Health* (New York: Gotham Books, 2004); Paul F. Campos, *The Diet Myth: Why America's Obsession with Weight Is Hazardous to Your Health* (New York: Gotham Books, 2005); Gard and Wright, *The Obesity Epidemic: Science, Morality, and Ideology*; Jan Wright and Valerie Harwood, *Biopolitics and the Obesity Epidemic: Governing Bodies* (London: Taylor & Francis, 2008); Gimlin, *Body Work: Beauty and Self-Image in American Culture*.

32 Marcia Millman, *Such a Pretty Face: Being Fat in America* (Toronto: Norton, 1980).

33 Richard Klein, *Eat Fat* (New York: Pantheon Books, 1996).

34 See, for example Rachel Colls' encounters with a club for fat women and men who have a sexual interest in them. Rachel Colls, "Big Girls Having Fun: Reflections on a 'Fat Accepting Space,'" *Somatechnics*, 2, no. 1 (2012): 18-37.

35 For example, Erdman Farrell appears unaware of high profile debates within the movement and misnames prominent activists. Erdman Farrell, *Fat Shame: Stigma and the Fat Body in American Culture*.

reveals NAAFA to other social scientists as a data source populated by compliant informants with a complicit management. Where NOLOSE[36] has gate-keeping strategies to protect its membership from exploitation by researchers and journalists, NAAFA does not. Erich Goode's sexual abuse of NAAFA members in the course of his ethnography of the organisation has not altered the organisation's stance, nor the willingness of researchers, including those who publicly criticised Goode, to use NAAFA as a study site.[37] His work continues to be cited as authoritative without comment about his problematic research tactics. More recently Jason Whitesel produced some of the fieldwork for his study whilst keeping his identity as a researcher stealth. He admits ethical concerns about this act, and recognises himself as a beneficiary of unearned thin privilege, but does not alter his working practices.[38]

A secondary proxy that has emerged from Millman's influential study, and which is present in many of the studies cited in this section, is that fat activism is primarily concerned with stigma. This is not to deny that stigma is an important site for fat activism. Erving Goffman's research into stigma influenced The Fat Underground's analysis of fat oppression, for example, and stigma is a common experience for fat people.[39] Samantha Thomas et al recognise that fat hatred has an impact on fat people but they treat this as a problem for individuals to overcome through the provision of anti-stigma campaigning, the details of which are nebulous

36 Also known informally as Fatlandia since 2010. NOLOSE, "Nolose.Org," http://www.nolose.org.
37 Erich Goode and J. Preissler, "The Fat Admirer." *Deviant Behavior,* 4 (1983): 175-202; Susan E. Bell, "Sexualizing Research: Response to Erich Goode," *Qualitative Sociology,* 25, no. 4 (2002): 535-39; Erich Goode, "Sexual Involvement and Social Research in a Fat Civil Rights Organization," *Qualitative Sociology,* 501-34; Abigail Saguy, "Sex, Inequality, and Ethnography: Response to Erich Goode," *Qualitative Sociology,* 24, no.4 (2002): 549-556.
38 Jason Whitesel, *Fat Gay Men: Girth, Mirth, and the Politics of Stigma* (New York: New York University Press, 2014).
39 Erving Goffman, *Stigma: Notes on the Management of Spoiled Identity* (London: Penguin, 1963); Sara Golda Bracha Fishman, "Life in the Fat Underground," http://www.radiancemagazine.com/issues/1998/winter_98/fat_underground.html; Cooper, *Fat & Proud: The Politics of Size.*

to say the least. They neglect to explore how fat activism might be part of a solution, that fat hatred is political, or even consider who might provide such anti-stigma work.[40] Meanwhile, a cluster of authors regard fat activism primarily as a strategic response to stigma.[41] Whilst it makes sense to develop a critical understanding of stigma, claiming that the primary goal of fat activism is to reduce stigma is also too reductive.

FAT ACTIVISM IS ABOUT EATING DISORDERS AND BODY IMAGE

In this proxy, fat activism is obscured by a feminist analysis of eating disorders; the politics of food; anti-dieting; beauty; body projects, including exercising and cosmetic surgery; and media. This influential work of Susie Orbach, Kim Chernin and Susan Bordo dominates public discussion about fat, gender and bodies to the extent that one might take it to represent the last feminist word on the subject.[42] But fat activism is

40 Samantha Thomas et al, "'Just Bloody Fat!': A Qualitative Study of Body Image, Self-Esteem and Coping in Obese Adults," *International Journal of Mental Health Promotion*, 12, no. 1 (2010): 39-49.

41 Marissa Dickins et al, "The Role of the Fatosphere in Fat Adults' Responses to Obesity Stigma: A Model of Empowerment without a Focus on Weight Loss," *Qualitative Health Research* 21, no. 12 (2011): 1679-91; Abigail C. Saguy and Anna Ward, "Coming out as Fat: Rethinking Stigma," *Social Psychology Quarterly,* 74 (2011): 53-75; Farrell Erdman, *Fat Shame: Stigma and the Fat Body in American Culture*; Jenny Ellison, "Weighing In: The 'Evidence of Experience' and Canadian Fat Women's Activism," *Canadian Bulletin of Medical History / Bulletin canadien d'histoire de la médecine,* 30, no. 1 (2013): 55-75; Whitesel, *Fat Gay Men: Girth, Mirth, and the Politics of Stigma*; Ngaire Donaghue, "The Moderating Effects of Socioeconomic Status on Relationships between Obesity Framing and Stigmatization of Fat People," *Fat Studies: An Interdisciplinary Journal of Body Weight and Society,* 3, no. 1 (2014): 6-16.

42 Orbach, *Fat Is a Feminist Issue*; Susie Orbach, *Fat Is a Feminist Issue 2: How to Free Yourself from Feeling Obsessive About Food* (London: Hamlyn, 1982); Susie Orbach, *Bodies* (London: Profile Books, 2009); Kim Chernin, *The Obsession: Reflections on the Tyranny of Slendernes* (New York: Harper & Row, 1981); Kim Chernin, *Womansize: The Tyranny of Slenderness* (London: The Women's Press, 1983); Kim Chernin, *The Hungry Self: Women, Eating and Identity*; Susan Bordo, *Unbearable Weight: Feminism, Western Culture, and the Body*, 10th anniversary ed (Berkeley, CA: University of California Press, 2003). See also Wendy Chapkis and Naomi Wolf, *Beauty Secrets: Women and the Politics of Appearance* (London: The Women's Press, 1986); Naomi Wolf, *The Beauty*

absent, the movement that I describe in this book has been completely
overlooked by these feminists.

The theoretical content of *Fat Is a Feminist Issue* has been critiqued
elsewhere for stereotyping and pathologising fat and upholding an ideal
of thinness.[43] Orbach and her colleagues at The Women's Therapy Centre
have denied these claims, arguing that they have been misinterpreted.[44]
At the time of its publication, fat activists in the US argued that the
stereotyping of fat in the book is because it does not engage with fat
people's experiences of fat oppression, and that it reproduces the problems
of being fat as medical and psychological rather than a result of the
political positioning of fat people.[45] British fat activists later reiterated
this position.[46] In 2009 Orbach acknowledged her support for fat feminist
activism at an Association of Size Diversity and Health conference,[47] but
in her work *Bodies*, published in the same year, she wrote in support of
anti-obesity policy.[48] Corinna Tomrley remarks:

Myth (London: Chatto, 1990) and works influenced by this such as Carol Munter
and Valerie Mason-John, "Fat and the Fantasy of Perfection" in *Pleasure and Danger:
Exploring Female Sexuality*, edited by Carole S. Vance, 225-31 (London: Pandora Press,
1992); Valerie Mason-John, "Keeping up Appearances: The Body and Eating Habits" in
Assaults on Convention: Essays on Lesbian Transgressors, edited by Nicola Godwin et al,
64-79 (London: Cassell, 1996). Indeed, in her critique of *Fat Is A Feminist Issue*, Cath
Jackson asks: "Why is it that women who haven't even read it assume it is a politically
sound analysis of women and bodysize?" Cath Jackson, "Fast Food Feminism," *Trouble
and Strife*, 7 (1985): 39-44.

43 Nicky Diamond, "Thin Is the Feminist Issue," *Feminist Review*, 19 (1985): 45-64;
Jackson, "Fast Food Feminism"; Cooper, *Fat & Proud: The Politics of Size*; Corinna
Tomrley, "Introduction: Finding the Fat, the Fighting and the Fabulous, Or: The Political,
Personal and Pertinent Imperatives of Fsuk," in *Fat Studies in the UK*, edited by Corinna
Tomrley and Ann Kaloski Naylor, 9-16 (York: Raw Nerve, 2009).

44 Susie Orbach and Compulsive Eating Supervision Study Group at The Women's
Therapy Centre, "Responses to Nicky Diamond," *Feminist Review*, 21 (1985): 119-22.

45 Helen Lizard and Shan, "Letter: Thin Thinking," *Off Our Backs*, 9, no. 5 (1979): 28;
Elly Janesdaughter, "Letter: Fatophobic Feminists," *Off Our Backs*, no. 7; Aldebaran
(Vivian Mayer), "Letter: Compulsive Eating Myth," *Off Our Backs*.

46 Tina Jenkins and Heather Smith, "Fat Liberation," *Spare Rib* 182 (1987): 14-18.

47 Association for Size Diversity and Health, *Susie Orbach*, Asdah National Conference.
Marriott, Dulles VA, 2009.

48 Orbach, *Bodies*.

What is so problematic about this is that she and her work – particularly *Fat is a Feminist Issue* are often portrayed as really, really important. Her work is undoubtedly influential. But I really think it's the idea of *FIFI* [*Fat is a Feminist Issue*] that has the influence a lot of the time, rather than what she actually wrote. Although the idea that women 'eat their feelings' and are hiding in fat is a pervasive one and came right out of that book. *FIFI* is considered an essential text for women to read and this is so scary. It's basically a diet book that pretends not to be a diet book so it has the potential to be really appealing to women for whom the words "she mentioned a woman who had lost lots of weight without dieting" and "I lost lots of weight" are magical and seductive. It's so, so flawed but gets reissued again and again. And each time Orbach writes a new intro appropriating fat activist speech yet says we're a problem all over again. She has not changed her tune, or retracted anything.[49]

Fat activism is relevant in many other fields and discourses, for example of the body, of embodied difference, embodied subjectivity, of health and illness, of gender, disability, ageing, citizenship and so on. Fat embodiment[50] is one of many intersections of marginalised identity through which people are socially constructed and situated. Given the use of intersectional analyses to theorise identity politics it is not surprising that fat is allied with other identity-based movements, particularly those that place the body centrally.[51] There are fruitful discussions to be had about all of these subjects and their relationships to each other. In 1988 in the US a coalition between a NAAFA Research Committee and the National Organisation of Women led to the establishment of the Body Image Task Force, which was an attempt to draw out these broader

49 Charlotte Cooper, "Rad Fatty: Corinna Tomrley." http://www.obesitytimebomb.blogspot.co.uk/2009/07/rad-fatty-corinna-tomrley.html.
50 Embodiment means how people experience their bodies.
51 Dawn Atkins, ed. *Looking Queer: Body Image and Identity in Lesbian, Bisexual, Gay, and Transgender Communities* (Binghampton, NY: The Haworth Press, Inc., 1998).

connections.[52] More recently The Body Is Not An Apology has developed this discussion.[53] But this has also transformed the discourse into one of body image rather than fat activism or fat feminism. It is my wish to make fat feminist activism explicit here as a subject in its own right. At the moment, the proxy has taken over, it has been falsely universalised, and the specificities of fatness or fat activism have been overlooked or lost.

FAT ACTIVISM IS ABOUT OBESITY AND HEALTH

Obesity discourse is totalitarian, by which I mean it presents itself as the only authority on fat, nothing else counts. Fat is a crisis brought about by a mismanagement of energy balance, it offers nothing of value, it is only an opportunity for intervention. It is always about health, and health is presented as an apolitical fact. As Aldebaran points out:

> Problems of fat people are not seen as political problems, but as medical problems; and not as needing a political solution but as needing a medical solution.[54]

Obesity is a stunningly limited frame for all the things that constitute being fat that are lumped together within it. Within this system fat activism is either ignored or presented as something illegitimate and ridiculous.

Foresight Tackling Obesities: Future Choices is a report that has greatly influenced UK government obesity policy and is a classic example of state-sponsored fatphobic tub-thumping. It is unusual in that it mentions the existence of fat activism, which it pegs as a response to stigma, although ironically the report fails to acknowledge that it might be reproducing such fat hatred. The reference is very slight, the authors

---

52 Cooper, *Fat & Proud: The Politics of Size.*
53 Taylor, "The Body Is Not an Apology."
54 Stein and Hoffstein, *Proceedings of the First Feminist Fat Activists' Working Meeting: April 18-20, 1980, New Haven, Ct.*

refer to fat activism as "'fat and proud' movements in the USA" and sandwich it in with some unrelated anti-obesity rhetoric.[55] This passage demonstrates how, even when a critical perspective is allowed to surface, it is instantly smothered by an obesity discourse that cannot account for it within an energy-balance model pathologising fatness. Here, the mis-named 'fat and proud'[56] movement is suggested as a response to a discourse of appearance, or an inexplicable normalising of the monstrous, and is situated only in the US. The citation is left hanging with no further examination and, of all the resources this massively-financed research[57] could use, a footnote offers a link to an obscure and out-dated website lacking any substance, which further implies that fat activism is of trifling consequence.[58] This is likely no accident. Abigail Saguy demonstrates how proponents of obesity discourse refuse to acknowledge fat activism or critical views because of their prejudice; this is not a case of being able to listen to evidence, it is a matter of maintaining power and status.[59]

Ironically, research based on obesity discourse is unlikely to be experienced by fat people, including activists, as emancipatory or health-enhancing. My own emotional response to such work encompasses feelings of powerlessness, anger that ranges from disgruntlement to rage and bewilderment at the flattening of the complexities of my life.

55 Bryony Butland et al, *Foresight Tackling Obesities: Future Choices–Project Report* (London: Government Office for Science, 2005).

56 I am interested in how 'fat and proud' is sometimes used as a shorthand for fat activism because of the title of my first book. This is not a term that people within the movement generally use to describe or name what they do or who they are. Elsewhere it has been derided. L Brooks, "Size Matters," http://www.shelleybovey.com/frameset.html?/sizematters.html. I sometimes wonder if my work has come to represent a proxy of fat activism to those who are invested in shutting it down.

57 For some years I have been struggling without success to get a Freedom of Information report on the public cost of Foresight's obesity research in order to compare it to claims about the public cost of fat people.

58 "Ringsurf: Fat and Proud." http://www.ringsurf.com/ring/fat_prd/.

59 Abigail Saguy, *What's Wrong with Fat?* (New York: Oxford University Press, 2014). This power is evident in Judy Freespirit's comments, paraphrased by Aldebaran: "Almost any fat woman who has lived a life of dieting is a creation in one way or another of the medical profession." Stein and Hoffstein, *Proceedings of the First Feminist Fat Activists' Working Meeting: April 18-20, 1980, New Haven, Ct.*

Physiological effects are congruent with stress: shallow breathing, a tight chest, a sinking feeling. These are encounters with systemic sanctioned hatred. Reading this work as a fat person requires a certain steeliness, it can be physically and emotionally depleting.

Not surprisingly, weight loss corporations have tended to stonewall fat activism, but Jennifer Grossman, then director of Dole's Nutrition Institute, which markets weight loss, published a sarcastic ethnography of a NAAFA Convention.[60] She argued that weight loss is the only viable means of overcoming fat hatred, which she would do because she has vested interests in selling this idea. Other dismissals are bound by ideology. Michael Fumento, neoconservative sceptic and corporate lackey, attacks fat activism because it is based on "bad science," as opposed to his own brand of quackery.[61] Fat activism has been dismissed in a similar vein by rationalists and through online hate fora, websites and social media.[62]

Scholars of the body who attempt to make sense of fat activism without sufficiently challenging obesity discourse tend to end up in a bit of a

60 Jennifer Grossman, "The Perils of 'Fat Acceptance,'" *National Review*, 55, no. 22 (2003): 34-38.

61 Michael Fumento, *The Fat of the Land: The Obesity Epidemic and How Overweight Americans Can Help Themselves* (New York: Viking/Allen Lane, 1997); Gard and Wright, *The Obesity Epidemic: Science, Morality, and Ideology*. One wonders what Fumento might have made of fat activists who share his political beliefs such as the *Big Liberty* RSS feed, which aggregates a number of libertarian fat activist blogs, or the work of Sandy Swarc, a blogger who is critical of the science of obesity as well as climate change. Big Liberty, "The Fat Liberation Feed," http://biglibertyblog.com/the-fat-liberation-feed/; Sandy Swarc, "Junkfood Science," http://junkfoodscience.blogspot.com/. He also shares much in common with Basham et al, *Diet Nation: Exposing the Obesity Crusade* (London: Social Affairs Unit, 2006).

62 RationalWiki, "Fat Acceptance Movement," http://rationalwiki.org/wiki/Fat_acceptance_movement; Anonymous, "Notyourgoodfatty.Com," http://notyourgoodfatty.com/; Reddit, "Removing Harassing Subreddits," http://np.reddit.com/r/announcements/comments/39bpam/removing_harassing_subreddits/. Kath Read writes extensively about being trolled on her blog Kath Read, "Fat Heffalump," https://fatheffalump.wordpress.com.

pickle.[63] Nick Crossley's take on the subject is typically abysmal.[64] He presents fat, as though it could be separated from people, as a social construction but reiterates it as fact, as epidemic, as crisis and energy balance. Some of his claims are understandable given the dearth of material available, but the rest of his discussion verges on the bizarre: only fat people support fat activism; Mama Cass is an icon of the movement[65]; "Fat Underground" is referenced in parenthesis with no explanation as to what it means, or even that it was an organisation. Crossley mentions that he has unearthed evidence about fat activism but does not cite any of it, nevertheless he mansplains authoritatively that the movement is "very limited".[66]

This is not to say that feminist academics who use obesity to explore fat activism are any better! Elspeth Probyn condemns it without a basic understanding of the subject.[67] She argues that fat activism keeps people fat, unhealthy and catastrophically consuming "cheap and bad products," the classism of which is common in origin stories ascribed to fat people.[68] She says it is imperative that feminists act against the global obesity epidemic, and denounces fat activism as some kind of cult. Antronette Yancey et al make similar arguments, and Lauren Berlant uses fatness as a metaphor for slow death, reproducing the tired clichés of fat people as pathological and morbid without sufficiently queering those states.[69]

---

63 Bryan S. Turner, *The Body and Society: Explorations in Social Theory*, 2nd ed. (London: SAGE Publications Ltd., 1996); Nick Crossley, "Sociology and the Body" in *The Sage Handbook of Sociology*, edited by Craig Calhoun et al (London: SAGE, 2005); Chris Shilling, *The Body and Social Theory*, 2nd ed. (London: SAGE, 1993).

64 Nick Crossley, "Fat Is a Sociological Issue: Obesity Rates in Late Modern, 'Body-Conscious' Societies," *Social Theory & Health* 2 (2004): 222-53.

65 Kind of true, but she's been dead for about 40 years.

66 Crossley, "Fat Is a Sociological Issue," 248. Similarly, fat activism is a major omission in Sander Gilman's cultural history of fat. Sander Gilman, *Fat: A Cultural History of Obesity* (Boston: Polity, 2008).

67 Elspeth Probyn, "Silences Behind the Mantra: Critiquing Feminist Fat," *Feminism & Psychology*, 18, no. 3 (2008): 401-04.

68 Probyn, "Silences Behind the Mantra: Critiquing Feminist Fat," 402.

69 Antronette K. Yancey et al, "Obesity at the Crossroads: Feminist and Public Health Perspectives," *Signs* 31, no. 2 (2006): 425-47; Lauren Berlant, "Slow Death (Sovereignty,

Less contentiously, there have been a number of studies using frame analysis to understand how fat is constructed in different social spaces, for example through organisations or philosophies.[70] This is a social science method of exploring how different people understand a subject, perhaps in contradictory or conflicting ways, and compare core beliefs or approaches of equivalent groups of people. The use of frame analysis undermines the idea that fat is a fixed scientific fact rather than a social construction and is hence a useful means of addressing the dominance of obesity discourse, which often draws on an idea of science and 'truth' that is beyond critique. Scholars compare weight loss organisations with fat activist organisations as if they were the same kind of thing, for example, or medicalised models with fat rights models. The problem with this is that these frames are presented as equal and distinct, and obesity and fat are conflated. Only Saguy refers to the overlaps between them and to the idea that some frames are more dominant and powerful than others.[71] I am wary of these analyses because they continue to use proxies for fat activism without much interrogation and this is too simplistic. For example, Saguy uses the concepts HAES, Beauty and Fat Rights to encompass much of fat activism but, as I will show, fat activism is not just a matter of health, beauty or seeking rights. She includes references

Obesity, Lateral Agency)" *Critical Inquiry* 33 (2007): 754-80.

70 Jeffrey Sobal and Donna Maurer, *Interpreting Weight: The Social Management of Fatness and Thinness* (Edison, NJ: Aldine Transaction, 1999); Jeffrey Sobal and Donna Maurer, *Weighty Issues: Fatness and Thinness as Social Problems* (Edison, NJ: Aldine Transaction, 1999); Daniel D. Martin, "From Appearance Tales to Oppression Tales: Frame Alignment and Organizational Identity," *Journal of Contemporary Ethnography* 31, no. 2 (2002): 158-206; Stefan Sturmer et al, "The Dual-Pathway Model of Social Movement Participation: The Case of the Fat Acceptance Movement," *Social Psychology Quarterly* 66, no. 1 (2003): 71-82; Saguy and Riley, "Weighing Both Sides: Morality, Mortality, and Framing Contests over Obesity"; Sonya Brown, "An Obscure Middle Ground: Size Acceptance Narratives and Photographs of 'Real Women,'" *Feminist Media Studies* 5, no. 2 (2005): 237-60; Josée Johnston and Judith Taylor, "Feminist Consumerism and Fat Activists: A Comparative Study of Grassroots Activism and the Dove Real Beauty Campaign," *Signs: Journal of Women in Culture and Society* 33, no. 4 (2008): 941-66; Kwan, "Framing the Fat Body: Contested Meanings between Government, Activists, and Industry."

71 Saguy, *What's Wrong with Fat?*

to The Chubsters as an organisation that is pursuing rights, but as the originator of this now somewhat expired project I would argue that The Chubsters has very little to do with rights and is more orientated towards a queer anti-social or a world of fantasy. In addition, fat activism or self-acceptance appears at the far end of the matrix, as though it is a conclusion rather than an on-going, non-linear question.[72] I suspect that frame analysis reveals more about how organisations, philosophies or sociologists function than fat activism.

There is a critical literature of obesity which has responded to the terms set by the dominant discourse. Where it is mentioned in this work, fat activism exists within the limits that obesity has already set. This is because such critical work seeks to influence and change obesity discourse through counter-evidence and must be articulated within it to be intelligible.[73] Fat subjectivity and fat activism becomes reduced to discourses on health, discrimination and stigma, and becomes appropriated by professionals in the clinic and in the academy.[74]

72 Andrea E. Bombaka, "'Obesities': Experiences and Perspectives across Weight Trajectories," *Health Sociology Review* (2015): 1-14. See also the many uses of progression models of fat activism that begin in abjection and end in acceptance. Carol Wiley, *Journeys to Self-Acceptance: Fat Women Speak* (Freedom, CA: The Crossing Press, 1994); Courtney, "Size Acceptance as a Grief Process: Observations from Psychotherapy with Lesbian Feminists."

73 Tracy L. Tylka et al, "The Weight-Inclusive Versus Weight-Normative Approach to Health: Evaluating the Evidence for Prioritizing Well-Being over Weight Loss," *Journal of Obesity* (2014) doi:10.1155/2014/983495; Sigrún Daníelsdóttir et al, "Academy for Eating Disorders Guidelines for Childhood Obesity Prevention Programs," Academy for Eating Disorders, http://aedweb.org/web/index.php/23-get-involved/position-statements/90-aed-statement-on-body-shaming-and-weight-prejudice-in-public-endeavors-to-reduce-obesity-4; Linda Bacon at al, "Size Acceptance and Intuitive Eating Improve Health for Obese, Female Chronic Dieters," *Journal of the American Dietetic Association* 105, no. 6 (2005): 929-36; Bacon and Aphramor, "Weight Science: Evaluating the Evidence for a Paradigm Shift." I could go on, the question of whether or not fat is healthy underscores a massive amount of critical literature.

74 The special issue of *Narrative Enquiry in BioEthics* exploring the American Medical Association's decision to call obesity a disease is a good example of this process. By presenting articles that reference fat activism alongside those that valorise weight loss it shows scant understanding of the critical nature of fat activism to obesity discourse and instead assimilates it into the dominant narrative. James DuBois et al, eds. *Narrative Inquiry in Bioethics,* Volume 4, Number 2, (2014).

Kelly Brownell's work at Yale University's Rudd Centre for Food Policy and Obesity condemns obesity discourse in various ways but maintains support for weight management, it doesn't treat fat activism as a viable and less risky public health strategy.[75] This reproduces the idea that fat is an awkward and intractable problem instead of finding answers within it; fat activism's main value is limited to challenging prejudice or promoting health. Fat activists are almost never consulted and fat people are repeatedly positioned as failed subjects, typically constructed as absent, abstract, abject, anonymous and Othered,[76] passive patient-consumers in need of expert intervention.

Where this proxy invites social change, it does so from a limited position; at its most radical it is a means of accessing obesity power and transforming it from within, but it also threatens to uphold those structures. The side-lining and refusal to acknowledge fat activism is a power tactic. Following the sociologists Pierre Bourdieu and Nancy Fraser, Andrew Sayer identifies misrecognition as a refusal of the powerful to see, or recognise as valid, real, and worthy of attention, those who do not share their power.[77] Bourdieu argues that the powerful

75 Kelly D. Brownell et al, *Weight Bias: Nature, Consequences, and Remedies* (New York: Guildford Press, 2005). Saguy refers to an exchange with Brownell in which he admits that he uses anti-obesity rhetoric as a strategy for attracting attention and funding for his "important" work. Saguy, *What's Wrong with Fat?*

76 Other when capitalised here refers to a noun or a verb used to describe those who are different to you, or who are made different and therefore estranged from the dominant culture.

77 Pierre Bourdieu and Loïc Wacquant, "Language, Gender and Symbolic Violence" in *An Invitation to Reflexive Sociology*, edited by Pierre Bourdieu and Loïc Wacquant, 140-74 (Cambridge: Polity, 1992); Nancy Fraser, "Who Counts? Dilemmas of Justice in a Postwestphalian World," *Antipode* 41 (2009): 281-197; Nancy Fraser, "Injustice at Intersecting Scales: On 'Social Exclusion' and the 'Global Poor,'" *European Journal of Social Theory* 13, no. 3 (2010): 363-71; Andrew Sayer, "Misecognition: The Unequal Division of Labour and Contributive Justice" in *The Politics of Misrecognition*, edited by Simon Thompson and Majid Yar, 87-104 (Farnham: Ashgate, 2011). In addition, Susanne Brandheim's paper on misrecognition in critical weight studies (sic) is, ironically, an example of the misrecognition of fat activism by academics orientated towards obesity discourse. The author mis-names prominent activists and gatherings, fails to cite basic literature, presents long-defunct groups and media as current, and has a poor grasp of the movement or its potential spaces for liberation. Brandheim,

can interpret social phenomena as they please because it is not in their interests to engage otherwise, bell hooks adds that these interests are gendered, racialised and classed.[78] Paolo Freire asserts that the powerful misrecognise because they are incapable of doing otherwise.[79] Bourdieu and Fraser acknowledge that misrecognition is a form of symbolic violence, it is cultural erasure. This is what is going on here.

DEVELOPING FAT ACTIVIST RESEARCH

These proxies have come to dominate how people think of fat activism because the dismissal of fat activism as superficial, secondary to other issues, not useful or worthy of investigation means that there is little impetus to develop research around it. Fat activism remains a marginal subject even within Fat Studies. Where it is addressed, the focus is too narrow and frequently reiterates dominant cultural values in problematic ways. So far, most researchers working on fat activism have lacked the capacity and experience to explore the subject extensively. The scholarly literature of fat activism is currently dominated by normatively-sized researchers who do not have their own histories of fat activism or community ties. They may be research experts but they are not expert in being or knowing fat activists. Angharad E. Beckett argues that if you want to understand a social movement, in her case disability activism, it is not enough to try and theorise it using existing models, you need new approaches that reflect the content of that movement.[80] I agree.

"The Misrecognition Mind-Set: A Trap in the Transformative Responsibility of Critical Weight Studies."

78 bell hooks, *Teaching to Transgress: Education as the Practice of Freedom* (New York: Routledge, 1994); Pierre Bourdieu, "The Forms of Capital" in *Handbook of Theory and Research for the Sociology of Education*, edited by John Richardson, 241-58 (New York: Greenwood, 1986).

79 Paulo Freire, *Pedagogy of the Oppressed* (London: Penguin, 1970).

80 Angharad E. Beckett, "Understanding Social Movements: Theorising the Disability Movement in Conditions of Late Modernity," *The Sociological Review* 54, no. 4 (2006): 734-52.

Over the next few pages I will explain how I came to develop my own approach to researching fat activism in the hope of generating other kinds of community-based knowledge that puts fat people at the centre of its production.

STANDPOINT

Who researches fat people and who creates knowledge about fatness is important, and the proof of that is in the poor quality of the fat activist research literature that I've discussed above; the work suffers when a strong and extensive engagement with fat activist community is absent. On the other hand, the literature of fat activism by fat activists, as I have shown, has yet to develop a rigorous scholarship or research tradition.

Cat Pausé's blog post, *The Epistemology of Fatness*, asks a great question: who is allowed to know about fat?[81] Epistemology means ideas about how people come to know things. Pausé argues that fat epistemology is granted to obesity experts who are far removed from fat embodiment, whilst fat people's knowledge-sharing about their own bodies and lives is ignored or ridiculed.[82] Fat people are frequently positioned as "repositories of data, data that ultimately is believed to be the property of the researcher".[83] This maintains obesity 'expertise' and the power enshrined within it. Obesity silences fat people whereas alternative discourses that recognise our humanity are where we find voice.[84] Pausé maintains, as I do, the

81 Cat Pausé, "The Epistemology of Fatness," http://friendofmarilyn.com/2012/04/05/the-epistemology-of-fatness/.

82 Let's not forget that fat people do not always enjoy the benefits of rigorous methods or sound ethics in research. Lucy Aphramor, "Validity of Claims Made in Weight Management Research: A Narrative Review of Dietetic Articles," *Nutrition Journal* 9, no. 30 (2010): na; J. Eric Oliver, *Fat Politics: The Real Story Behind America's Obesity Epidemic* (New York: Oxford University Press US, 2006); Linda Bacon, *Health at Every Size: The Surprising Truth About Your Weight* (Dallas TX: BenBella Books, 2008).

83 Zoë C. Meleo-Erwin, "Fat Bodies, Qualitative Research and the Spirit of Participatory Action Research," *International Review of Qualitative Research* 3, no. 3 (2010): 335-50.

84 Jean Ochterski, "There Are No Fat People in the Netherlands: Embodied Identities,

imperative that epistemology derived from fat people's own experience must be taken seriously in order to know about fat and change how knowledge and power are currently used against fat people. But at present there is a gap between the objects and producers of knowledge.

Standpoint, a researcher's attitude and relationship to the research subject, tends to receive poor attention, perhaps a paragraph or sentence or two. It is not the basis of the work as it is here. Thinner researchers may argue that standpoint is not important, for example they might say that anyone can be fat enough or that fat and thin are false binaries. This looks similar to the fantasy of colour-blindness, an attempt not to acknowledge differences that matter for fear of revealing an imbalance of power. Deborah Lupton has criticised my belief that fat people should be agents of our own lives and central producers of knowledge about fat.[85] This does not mean that other people should not also write and think about fat because, as Lupton points out, obesity discourse negatively affects people of all sizes. But it means that fat people should be recognised as important knowledge producers and that academics and policy-makers of all sizes should support fat people in claiming space to produce that knowledge. 'Nothing About Us Without Us,' a slogan from the disability rights movement, perfectly captures the need for inclusion in knowledge production. Disabled and trans people and sex workers, not to mention the entire world beyond the dominant West, have struggled for fair representation and agency within a context where they are continuously spoken for by privileged experts removed from their day to day lives. This is an issue of challenging power and unquestioned entitlement to speak and of developing the self-determination of fat people.

It is painful to talk about these differences within research communities where there are many normatively-embodied practitioners and where fat people need their support, perhaps as supervisors, funding gate-keepers or colleagues. Speaking up exposes uncomfortable power relationships,

Hypervisibility, and the Contextual Relevancy of Fatness" in *Independent Study Project (ISP) Collection* (South Hadley, MA: Mount Holyoke College, 2013).
85 Deborah Lupton, *Fat* (Abingdon: Routledge, 2012).

it risks making fat researchers more invisible and marginal. It exposes privilege, authenticity and authority, and it may reveal instances where not being fat *does* negatively affect research. Megan Warin and Jessica Gunson conducted a small literature review about being normatively-embodied obesity researchers, they acknowledge that this produces silences in the research and affects what participants share.[86]

Carol Wiley's edited collection of interviews is often overlooked because of its methodological limitations, yet it may be the only example of a first person fat activist community ethnography that isn't built on internalised self-loathing.[87] This is not to say that only certain types of idealised self-loving fat people should research fat activism. Instead, it is a comment on the scarcity of work about fat activism by people who represent the possibility that self-hatred is not the only narrative for being fat. Research produced by fat activists who do not harbour desires to lose weight, present accounts of their own weight loss, or profess an intolerance of their own bodies, and who represent, even in part, the self-acceptance that is important to fat political movements remains rare. A number of authors who have written about fat, proxies for fat, and fat activism have talked about their fatness on a spectrum that stretches from deep horror to ambivalence, without addressing other possibilities for being fat.[88]

One's fatness and self-acceptance, or lack of it, shouldn't matter but at the moment the sheer paucity of work produced by those with direct experience of activism and of being fat means that it does matter. I do not want to suggest that there is a universal fat person who can claim to speak for all fat activists. Hannele Harjunen says that being fat gives one

---

86 Megan J. Warin and Jessica S. Gunson, "The Weight of the Word: Knowing Silences in Obesity Research," *Qualitative Health Research* XX, no. X (2013): 1-11.

87 Wiley, *Journeys to Self-Acceptance: Fat Women Speak.*

88 Bovey, *What Have You Got to Lose?*; Bordo, *Unbearable Weight: Feminism, Western Culture, and the Body*; Campos, *The Diet Myth: Why America's Obsession with Weight Is Hazardous to Your Health*; Samantha Murray, "'Banded Bodies': The Somatechnics of Gastric Banding" in *Somatechnics: Queering the Technologisation of Bodies*, edited by Nikki Sullivan and Samantha Murray, 153-70 (London: Ashgate, 2009).

access to certain kinds of knowing, which she calls "the fat experience".[89]
I am wary of this, however, because I think there is a danger that people's
differences concerning that experience will be ignored.

THEORIES

I am interested in supporting research that helps develop fat activism
and which is a result of the direct experiences of fat activists, especially
those who are fat and come from the margins. I understand this as a
valuable means of undoing the proxies that currently stand-in for fat
activism and helping to develop a more realistic view of the movement.
I want fat people to be prime instigators of fat epistemology and to
be respected as such. I hope this book goes some way in helping to
develop this idea. I think of the methodology for this study as part of
the project's activism because it proposes ways of knowing – tentative,
unorthodox, creative, emotive – that are a direct challenge to those
which predominate in obesity discourse. Methodology means not
only the methods that a researcher might use to gather information,
but the rationale for those methods. The rationale affects the kinds of
data and knowledge that arises from research. Theory supports the
rationale for research which in turn helps create methodology. I used
a handful of ideas to help shape the research.

Foucault, power, social movements

I started with the broad assumption that fat activism is about power and
agency. Michel Foucault's work on governmentality is commonly used to
theorise bodies in relation to power and has been used by people interested
in how fat people are socially controlled, stratified, surveilled, regimented,

---

89 Hannele Harjunen, *Women and Fat: Approaches to the Social Study of Fatness*,
Jyväskylä Studies in Education, Psychology and Social Research (Jyväskylä: Jyväskylän
Yliopisto, 2010).

patrolled, and self-governing.[90] Although governmentality accounts for the conditions from which fat activism might arise, it does not explain what it is that fat activists do. Indeed, by focusing on governmentality to the exclusion of other ideas about the uses of power that Foucault helpfully provides, the discourse of fat, including critical discourse, remains one of helplessness in the face of overwhelming social control.

A different reading of Foucault reveals that governmentality is a truncated analysis of power, it reveals the subtlety of power but it does not fully support the possibility of active resistance as a response to and as a kind of power in its own right. In *The History of Sexuality*, and elsewhere, power is not enshrined within authorities feeding down to the lowliest subject, it is a dynamic field in which everyone is implicated.[91] Resistance is always present because the relations of power generate numerous sites for action, so that a plurality of action occurs in relation to power. This is a helpful idea because it recognises that fat people are present and active in a field of power, which could be

90 Michel Foucault, *Discipline and Punish: The Birth of the Prison* (New York: Random House, 1977); Sandra Lee Bartky, "Foucault, Femininity and the Modernisation of Patriarchal Power" in *Feminism and Foucault: Paths of Resistance*, edited by Lee Quinby and Irene Diamond, 61-86 (Boston: Northeastern University Press, 1988); Bryan Turner, *Regulating Bodies: Essays in Medical Sociology* (London: Routledge, 1992); Elizabeth Grosz, *Volatile Bodies: Towards a Corporeal Feminism* (Bloomington, IN: Indiana University Press, 1994); Susan Bordo, "Feminism, Foucault and the Politics of the Body" in *Feminist Theory and the Body: A Reader*, edited by Janet Price and Margrit Shildrick, 246-57 (Edinburgh: Edinburgh University Press, 1999); John Evans et al, *Education, Disordered Eating and Obesity Discourse: Fat Fabrications* (Abingdon: Routledge, 2008); Bethan Evans and Rachel Colls, "Measuring Fatness, Governing Bodies: The Spatialities of the Body Mass Index (Bmi) in Anti-Obesity Politics," *Antipode: A Radical Journal of Geography* 41, no. 5 (2009): 1051-83; Kathryn Pauly Morgan, "Foucault, Ugly Ducklings, and Technoswans: Analysing Fat Hatred, Weight-Loss Surgery, and Compulsory Biomedicalised Aesthetics in America," *The International Journal of Feminist Approaches to Bioethics* 4, no. 1 (2011): 188-220; Heather Sykes, *Queer Bodies: Sexualities, Genders, & Fatness in Physical Education* (New York: Peter Lang, 2011).

91 Foucault, "Power and Strategies"; Foucault and Gordon, *Power/Knowledge: Selected Interviews and Other Writings, 1972-1977*; Michel Foucault, *The History of Sexuality, Vol. 1.* Harmondsworth: Penguin, 1981; Michel Foucault, "The Subject and Power" in *Michel Foucault: Beyond Structuralism and Hermeneutics*, edited by Hubert Dreyfus and Paul Rabinow (Chicago: University of Chicago Press, 1982).

named 'obesity' or 'fat,' and which shares turf with other fields of power. This field is not only about those presumed to exercise authority, but also other players who can no longer be discounted as an anonymous population that is merely 'done to'. What those other players do is what concerns me here.

The killjoy

Sara Ahmed has produced the figure of the feminist, queer and migrant killjoy to discuss how "happiness" is forced when things do not make allowances for pain, ambivalence, uneasiness, disruption and anger, or acknowledge oppression.[92] She argues that happiness is built on privilege, that it is those at the top of the pile who are the arbiters of what constitutes happiness, and those underneath expose that fiction through the role of the killjoy. In this context, the killjoy is a figure of resistance and integrity, someone who doesn't go along with things. In her essay *Axiomatic*, Eve Kosofsky Sedgwick writes of the power of the margins. She argues that people pushed to the margins, the ones who don't agree, the killjoys in other words, are also a part of the centre because it is from the margins that they disturb and disrupt the centre.[93] The margins are an important place to be. Unlike the popular literature of fat activism, and the scholarly literature that has failed to interrogate it sufficiently, I do not present fat activism as a happy endeavour of self-acceptance and healthy living; I do not offer it here as a cheery promise. Fat activism is much more complicated than that! The figure of the killjoy creates an opportunity to explore the phenomenon in-depth, to reformulate it, to be critical, and to do so as part of a displaced and marginal community.

Research Justice

92 Sara Ahmed, *The Promise of Happiness* (Durham, NC: Duke University Press, 2010).
93 Eve Kosofsky Sedgwick, "Axiomatic" in *Queer Theory*, edited by Iain Morland and Annabelle Willox, 81-95 (Basingstoke: Palgrave Macmillan, 2005).

The idea that marginalised communities benefit from the studies conducted about them and that research and researchers are held accountable is central to Research Justice, a methodological framework emerging through social justice and indigenous people's activism in the US.[94] This framework shares similar values to Participant (or Participatory) Action Research, which has already been proposed as a potential strategy for researching fat activism.[95] This is a useful model for fat activist-researchers conducting fat activist community research because of its commitment to ethical practice and harm minimisation, and because it invites critical reflection on the privilege, power and obligations of the researcher. But Research Justice extends this by acknowledging that research is political and treating it as a form of collaborative activism.[96] It is a bottom-up, not top down conceptualisation of knowledge production. It supports people's capacity to influence social policy and social change by developing confidence and skills in generating and legitimising community-based knowledge. This enables people to leverage power and negotiate with local, peer, mainstream or institutional knowledge producers. Research justice recognises the expertise and knowledge production methods of people in communities, drawn from indigenous practices, for example through conversation and oral testimonies.[97] It uses tactics such as open source publishing and translating work, training

94 Jeffrey P. Kahn et al, eds, *Beyond Consent: Seeking Justice in Research* (Oxford: Oxford University Press, 1998); Linda Tuhiwai Smith, *Decolonizing Methodologies: Research and Indigenous Peoples* (London: Zed Books, 1999); Allied Media Conference, *Research Justice for Movements and Community Voices*, edited by Allied Media Projects Detroit 2012; Reem Assil et al, "An Introduction to Research Justice," DataCenter, https://www.z2systems.com/np/clients/datacenter/product.jsp;jsessionid=2F1EEE41401FBEAD18A848DED1D302E7?product=5.

95 Meleo-Erwin, "Fat Bodies, Qualitative Research and the Spirit of Participatory Action Research."

96 Mastroiannim Kahn and Sugarman, *Beyond Consent: Seeking Justice in Research.* See my project "No More Stitch-Ups! Developing Media Literacy Through Fat Activist Community Research" for more in this vein. Charlotte Cooper, "No More Stitch-Ups: Media Literacy for Fat Activists," http://obesitytimebomb.blogspot.co.uk/2013/05/no-more-stitch-ups-media-literacy-for.html.

97 DataCenter, "Research Justice," http://www.datacenter.org/research-justice/.

in research methods or the use of community ethics committees. This study uses Research Justice to reconsider how fat people are positioned in obesity research and to shift us from passive, abjected objects, into active roles as reflective researchers, knowing research participants, activist-researcher-participants and owners of knowledge. I consider research here as a tool for building social movements and coalitions, and fostering community healing.

Scavenging qualitative methodology

Instead of following one particular research tradition to the letter, I adapted, customised and scavenged a mixture of research tactics for this study as a means of messing with or queering research. I wanted it to be qualitative, built on people's stories and my own experience with fat activism. It needed to be a *critical* ethnography, a means of challenging how fat people are socially constructed as research objects. I was influenced by Ben Agger, who states: "Methods make the reader believe that she is reading science and not fiction, but it is all fiction anyway".[98] I didn't want to present something as fact or truth, but rather my take on things. Because this work is about me and my context, it made sense to use an approach called autoethnography, where the researcher writes themselves into the work; they are part of the work, not a naïve outsider.[99] I am not the only fat person to employ this method.[100] Others patronise autoethnography as "radical

98 Ben Agger, "Does Postmodernism Make You Mad? Or, Did You Flunk Statistics?" in *The Sage Handbook of Social Science Methodology*, edited by William Outhwaite and Stephen P. Turner, 443-56 (Thousand Oaks, CA: SAGE Publications Inc., 2007).
99 Deborah E. Reed-Danahay, *Auto/Ethnography: Rewriting the Self and the Social* (Oxford: Berg, 1997); Amanda Coffey, *The Ethnographic Self: Fieldwork and the Representation of Identity* (London: SAGE, 1999); Carolyn Ellis, *The Ethnographic I: A Methodological Novel About Autoethnography* (Walnut Creek, CA: AltaMira Press, 2004); Heewon Chang, *Autoethnography as Method* (Walnut Creek, CA: Left Coast Press, 2008). I liked that Tami Spry described autoethnography as "academic heresy" – very punk! Tami Spry, "Performing Autoethnography: An Embodied Methodological Praxis" in *Emergent Methods in Social Research*, edited by Sharlene Nagy Hesse-Biber and Patricia Leavy, 183-211 (Thousand Oaks, CA: SAGE, 2006).
100 Sophie Smailes, "Negotiating and Navigating My Fat Body—Feminist

chic" but Tami Spry argues that it is powerful because it can destabilise researcher privilege, bring marginal experience to the centre, and provide "a mechanism for extending ethnography beyond the academy," a quality that has the potential to bring it in line with Research Justice.[101]

METHODS

Keeping theories of agency, critique, social justice and postmodern research techniques in mind, I developed a plan for how I would generate and treat the research data. What follows is an overview of the methods I used to research fat activism. This mostly involved doing activism, talking to fat activists in my social networks, and sifting through archival material.

Doing activism

I did fat activism and I thought about it critically. I have spent my adult life living in various states of financial precarity and my PhD funding was the first time that I could enjoy a secure income for four years. I took advantage of this to do as much fat activism as I could manage, to think about the different activities that I understood as activism and to broaden my repertoire. In 2011 my fat activism looked like this:

> My fat activism is pretty integrated into my life, it's not something that I need to put on a special outfit to perform or go to a particular place, so this means that it's just what I do every day. I can give some examples. Typically it might involve answering emails, lately I've been involved in a long and difficult exchange with an acquaintance who is on a diet and who got really angry when I

Autoethnographic Encounters," *Athenea Digital* 14, no. 1 (2014): 49-61.
101 Paul Atkinson et al, *Key Themes in Qualitative Research: Continuities and Change* (Walnut Creek, CA: Altamira Press, 2003); Spry, "Performing Autoethnography."

wrote a blog post criticising the company to which she is giving her time, energy and money. I'm writing a piece for a friend's zine about DIY[102] activism, and the fat consciousness we've both brought to that scene, and I'm also writing a Chubsters workshop plan for an event in March. The Chubsters is my semi-fictitious platform for all kinds of peculiar fat activism, and at this workshop we'll be learning how to behave in an anti-social way, learning how to spit accurately and to shoot spud guns! I'll also show a film I made about the gang and talk about its history. I'll make plans to attend a Fat Studies seminar later in the spring. I'll probably update my blog later today with some thoughts about hybridity and fat activist community belonging, though I'll try and make it sound less dry. I'll exchange quips on Facebook with other friends doing similar work, there's a fatshion (fat + fashion) blogger gathering at the weekend for example that's been organised online, maybe I'll Skype with a fat pal in California. I'll book a plane ticket to Hamburg, where I will be an Artist in Residence in a couple of months, making a zine out of a *Fat and Queer Trans Timeline* that I helped build and facilitate at a workshop last year, and finding out more about fat activism in Germany. I'll dance around my flat a bit, and I may go swimming. I'll post a cassette back to some older Jewish lesbian fat activists in Boston, they lent me a recording of two radio shows they produced in 1984 and 1985, my boyfriend digitised them and we are hoping to make them publicly available again, they are spectacular. I'll chat about some fat stuff I've been thinking about with my loves. I'll eat something good I've made and do some reading, I'm taking part in a reading series called *Race Revolt*, a kind of queer, anarchist activism on race and racism in the UK, and I'm interested in broadening my fat activism to include some of these ideas. Oh, and I'll do some work![103]

102 Do It Yourself, independent, cultural production. DIY has a strong relationship with punk and includes forms such as zines, alternative distribution networks, and performance subcultures.
103 Hannele Harjunen, "Normality Is Overrated," *NormiHomoLehti* (2011): 16-19.

Talking to fat activists

I wanted this work to reflect fat activist community so I conducted 31 interviews with people from my social networks. By social network I mean people related to me through friendship and political, social and sexual kinship. I was able to find people because of my fat activism. These networks are often maintained online because of geographical distance. The relationships within this social network sample varied: some participants knew each other, some were intimates of mine and of each other, some were more distant and isolated. I met two contributors for the first time during the interviewing period, and another is an acquaintance I have yet to meet offline.

During the sampling stage I defined 'fat activist' as people who do a broad range of activities that address fatness with a critical edge, who bring a consciousness to those activities, and who see themselves as part of a movement. I was particularly interested in queer and trans fat activists because of the ideas I was developing about genealogies of the movement. This is a form of theory-based sampling. I relied on opportunistic sampling, looking for intensity rich cases, and sequential sampling, a quality assurance strategy to expand the sampling frame and address issues and themes that arose during the data gathering period. Despite their extensive knowledge and experience of fat activism, there were some people I did not approach to interview because I don't have much of a rapport or relationship with them. This omission highlights some of the tensions that exist within fat activism, it exposes the myth of convivial homogeneity that I will explore later.

I included one participant who did not regard themselves as a fat activist as a disconfirming case regarding fat activist identity in the sample. I wanted to consider if whether or not one calls oneself a fat activist mattered; I wondered if what one does could be called fat activism if one does not identify as an activist. Can only self-identified fat activists call what they do fat activism? According to this disconfirming case it does not matter. During the interview the participant and I talked about this, we reflected that some of her work could be regarded as fat activism, and she experimented in calling herself a fat activist. This person did not fit the pattern in the sample but her inclusion in the sample enriched the idea of 'fat activist' and 'fat activism'. Some forms of activism are well-represented in this sample, and some less so, for example many participants referenced NOLOSE but few mentioned BBW[104] subcultures because these do not tend to attract a queer constituency.

The sample was located in the UK, Germany, the US, Canada, and Australia. One participant is from Finland but was interviewed outside their native country. All the participants lived in cities ranging from capitals to county seats. The sample was limited to my networks, and reflects a bias towards Western Anglophone subcultures, though two participants were bilingual, and English was not the first language for one person. It also reflects a bias towards educational status since all but two of the sample had been to university. The youngest participant was in their twenties, the oldest was close to seventy years old, with a mean[105] age of 35. The sample identified mostly as women, and also included five people who described themselves as trans and genderqueer. All but one of the sample was queer. Five were disabled. Two participants described themselves as people of colour, two came from mixed racial and ethnic backgrounds, another ten were members of minority ethnic groups, including Jews of Ashkenazi and Sephardic descent. Two of the participants stated religious affiliations. A number of class subject positions were represented in the sample, slightly more middle- than working class, with three people from upper middle class backgrounds. Five were single, the rest were in relationships of which four were non-monogamous. Four were parents. The sample ranged from smaller-fat to supersize.[106] There was an equal distribution of participants regarding their experience of fat activism over a period of time; some were relatively new to the movement, some were seasoned activists and some had many

---

104   Big Beautiful Women, a fat subculture.

105   Mean is a way of expressing average. All the ages were added together and divided by the number of participants.

106   Superfat or supersize are fat community terms for the fattest fat people.

years to draw on. It is possible that I missed cues around identity, and people may have said less to me than they would have said to a peer of a similar background. However, even with its limitations, this research was unusual in presenting and acknowledging this diverse a group of fat activist participants in qualitative research. Only one of the sample represented a dominant culture white, middle class, cis, heterosexual, able-bodied demographic. Seeking out a mixture of fat activist identities was an attempt to challenge the idea of a unified or universal fat activist voice and present fat activists as intersectional beings who exist in multiple contexts.[107]

There were many more people that I wanted to interview than I could manage. On reflection, I could have sampled many more older participants and people of colour as well as those with experience of fat activism in New York in the 1990s, where there was an active scene. I was unable to find Irish fat activists because my social networks in Ireland, where the PhD was based, were not well-developed enough. The same goes for fat activists beyond the West. It would have been interesting to include material from Bears[108] to bring in a different kind of non-feminist queer fat culture. I omitted other parties who are implicated in fat activism, for example people constructed as allies. Talking to a sample of people who do fat activism does not say much about those who witness it, or about the reception or understanding of fat activism amongst non-activists. It is beyond the scope of this research to explore those subjects but these ideas could be developed later.

I completed the interviews between June 2010 and January 2011, including a pilot study in the Bay Area. This breaks down as 22 face-to-face and Skype interviews, the eight face-to-face pilot interviews, and one email interview. Everybody I approached agreed to participate,

---

107 Ngaire Donaghue's paper on framing fat is a reminder that fat people are understood differently in different spaces and places. Donaghue, "The Moderating Effects of Socioeconomic Status on Relationships between Obesity Framing and Stigmatization of Fat People."

108 A gay sexual and social subculture focused on the convergence of masculinity and the body, including those bodies that are fat and/or hairy.

although scheduling conflicts prevented interviews with two prospective participants. The interviews were unstructured, like conversations, a process of co-creation.[109] I used interviews instead of participant observation because participants would be more likely to be focused and present, not caught unawares and my process would be transparent. I excluded private details that I knew about people through our prior relationships and used only what participants told me in the interview, or in public and published sources. I was explicit in the written consent form about what I would and would not share and was as clear as I could be about my intentions for the research. I remain invested in continuing relationships with people who supported this work beyond the boundaries of the study. I feel a great responsibility to the participants.

When all of the interviews were over, I transcribed and analysed them using a grounded theory approach. This meant sifting through the transcripts looking for themes, patterns and comments that piqued my curiosity and building up a picture of fat activism directly from these community voices. I was drawn in particular to: what people did as fat activism and how they thought about it; conversations where people's experiences of fat activism contravened or was more sophisticated than published accounts; what fat activist community looked like to this group; corroborated information about historical events and interventions; and how participants felt and thought about feminism and queer theory.

I used this information to determine the content of this book and have included parts of the interview transcripts to keep a sense of the conversations and relationships from which these ideas have sprung. Some of the chapters have fewer interview quotes in them, particularly in places where the material is based on the research of reading secondary sources and encountering archival material, or my theorising of the movement. Long gaps between writing up my research as a thesis and as a book gave me more opportunities to reflect on what people did and

109 Barbara Sherman Heyl, "Ethnographic Interviewing" in *Handbook of Ethnography*, edited by Paul Atkinson et al, 369-83 (London: SAGE Publications Ltd, 2001).

didn't say during the interviewing period in 2010-2011. When there were quotations available to illustrate a point, I have used them, but these were not always available. Sometimes what was absent enabled me to develop my ideas, for example the poverty of fat activist historicising[110] or the lack of theorising fat activism.

I have used pseudonyms and altered identifying details to protect participants' anonymity in all cases, except for Judy, who died during the production of this work. Judy's private journals and papers are available in public archives and in death I felt that she no longer needed the protection of anonymity. But for the others I felt that anonymity would enable people to feel safe in sharing their thoughts with me and the readers of my work. I was grateful that people had agreed to speak to me on the record and I continue to feel strongly that their accounts represent a vital breaking of silence around fat people's self-representation. Where participants said things that challenged me, I have tried to incorporate their comments respectfully. I felt protective towards fat activists, I did not want to jeopardise anybody's safety in a context where all of us are under constant social attack in one form or another.

The University of Limerick Research Ethics Committee approved this study on the basis of it doing no harm, offering as much informed consent as possible, and having strong confidentiality procedures and data protection. In order to maintain the quality of the research, I kept my supervisors informed as it progressed and solicited feedback from them, as well as from peers and participants. As the thesis was turned into a book I continued to seek comments and criticism from other fat activists. I openly shared and developed concepts and arguments relating to the research through blogging, participation in events, presentations, and through invitations to speak. I offered my work and skills to other activists and researchers. I understood this as part of the process of being accountable to the study participants and communities of which I am a part, creating opportunities for feedback and developing my sensitivity to anti-oppressive practice.

---

110 Historicising means understanding the historical significance of something.

It would have been helpful for me formalise the question of why people agreed to be interviewed. Some offered their own reasons, unasked, such as wanting to support fat activism, or wanting to help me because we are friends, or wanting to talk about fat activism with me, but the issue of reciprocity was not always explicit. It would be a mistake to sidestep the issue of who this work serves. This research is likely to bring me some social capital and a small amount of money and is based on data that people have given for free. My involvement with fat activism has also entailed years of unpaid and far less recognised work, which I continue to do. In addition, there is plenty that I do not get out of this project. Trashing, social exclusion and a lot of stress are facts of life for activist-researchers working with their own communities and this has been part of my experience in producing this book. Negotiating research ethics, relationships and accountability has not been easy. Friendships ended with some of the people who participated in the study and these losses were experienced as personally and professionally devastating. There were other community fractures and personal struggles that made the work difficult to do. As Julia Downes, Maddie Breeze and Naomi Griffin point out, researchers are rarely prepared for these challenges, me included.[111]

Using and thinking about archives

Doing autoethnography helped me to reconsider the research space that is usually referred to as 'The Field.' This is usually a place that can be entered and left by ethnographers who retreat and write up their research elsewhere. I wanted to put aside the issue of 'going native,' a troubling term with colonial implications, to think instead about what the field means to somebody for whom it is not separate to everyday life. The autoethnographer Carolyn Ellis proposes the field is a series of spaces and strategies, "everything you do to gather information in

---

111 Julia Downes et al, "Researching Diy Cultures: Towards a Situated Ethical Practice for Activist-Academia," *Graduate Journal of Social Science* 10, no. 3 (2013).

a setting," which helped me to think of the field as a series of potential spaces where things happen.[112]

For me, as well as doing activism and interviewing people, the field in this sense ended up looking like an archive. I sought out archives that had holdings of historical fat activist material during the period in which I was collecting data. I wanted to place my experience of fat activism within historical contexts and needed primary material that is generally hard to find because of a lack of secondary documentation. So I travelled to three archives in the US, three in the UK, two in Germany, and sifted through a handful of online archives. I searched for fat activism in autonomous feminist and anarchist spaces in the UK and Australia, particularly those that had zine[113] libraries.

Working in the archive was not only illuminating with regard to gathering historical materials, it was a very emotional and inspiring experience. This is not surprising, Ann Cvetkovich points out that archives are potent spaces for queer activists because they highlight the public importance of private lives, the ephemeral is afforded some permanency, and there is potential for transforming the trauma of marginalisation.[114] How could I not feel overwhelmed, awed, delighted, or empowered by evidence of queer feminist fat activism given how it has been consistently disregarded or belittled? The archives became places of refuge and affirmation for me. It felt as though I was visiting a faraway yet familiar place, it put me in touch with past lives, people I knew vaguely and past instances of my own activism. I was able to watch a rare video of fat activists in the early 1970s, to see some of the people I'd only been able to read about previously, people who were heroic to me. I read Judy Freespirit's diaries. From time to time I would come across my own work that either I, or others, had donated. I felt very much that I was part of something bigger than myself, and this enabled me to

---

112 Ellis, *The Ethnographic I: A Methodological Novel About Autoethnography.*

113 A small scale, sometimes homemade, independent publication.

114 Ann Cvetkovich, *An Archive of Feelings: Trauma, Sexuality, and Lesbian Public Cultures* (Durham, NC: Duke University Press, 2003).

think of fat feminism and fat activism as entities that travel and shift over space and time.

I considered online fat activism within the text where it is relevant, but have not produced substantive work on this kind of activism as a distinct category or treated it as a field in its own right. This is for three reasons: first, online activism and the evolution of the Fatosphere is a massive subject in itself and there are a number of Fat Studies scholars who are already producing work in this area.[115] Secondly, there are currently a limited number of feeds, a system of gathering blog content, which makes it difficult to map the extent of the Fatosphere. Feeds, such as *Notes From the Fatosphere* and *Fat Chat*, reflect the tastes of their curators and tend to lean towards health, popular culture and fatshion from writers based in the US, with hardly any material that extends beyond these popular discourses. This represents a fraction of online activity relating to fat activism, which has rich cultures in social networking, through micro-blogging sites and other forms of creative or specialist social networks which are beyond the reach of such feeds. Thirdly, the online activism could be regarded as a discrete category, but the internet is embedded in the daily lives of the sample. With this in mind, I have chosen to treat online activism as another kind of activity rather than a special case.

When I reflect on the richness of the material that I was able to gather during this research project I realise how much methodology matters. The methods I used, and the ideas behind them, enabled me to create a far more detailed picture of what fat activists do than I had been able to find in popular and scholarly literature on the subject. I will explain these findings in the following chapters. Not only that, but my methodology implicitly challenges obesity research ethics and the overreliance

---

115 Dickins et al, "The Role of the Fatosphere in Fat Adults' Responses to Obesity Stigma: A Model of Empowerment without a Focus on Weight Loss"; Adwoa A. Afful and Rose Ricciardelli, "Shaping the Online Fat Acceptance Movement: Talking About Body Image and Beauty Standards," *Journal of Gender Studies* 24, no. 3 (2015): 1-20; Carolyn Bronstein, "Fat Acceptance Blogging, Female Bodies and the Politics of Emotion," *Feral Feminisms* no. 3 (2015): 106-18.

on top-down 'hard' medicalised science as the only possible way of constructing knowledge about fat people. Inexpensive community-based studies like my own reveal a lot about what fat people actually need and want and this piece of work suggests that researchers who disengage with the agency of fat people, or who ignore fat activist community, do so at their own peril.

DOING

I have described a series of fragments that are generally understood to represent fat activism as a whole. Fat activism is self-acceptance, it's about being body positive, it's campaigning for social change, it's challenging stigma, it's about eating, it's about health, it's negligible. But I have argued that these are merely proxies for a movement that is much more expansive and sophisticated than it has been given credit for. These proxies try to simplify a social phenomenon that cannot be reduced or contained, as I will now show.

In this chapter I present the findings to my basic research question: what is fat activism? I think of it being potentially limitless but here I will discuss some of the forms that the research sample shared with me. These include political process activism, which means the kind of things that most people in the West think of as activism; community-building; cultural work; micro fat activism, which takes place in very small social spaces; and ambiguous activism.

I am excited to show people what some fat activists actually do because there is a vast gulf between how fat activism is written about and how it is produced. Instead of trying to restrict what they do, fat activists might relish the sprawling, unruly, indefinable project they have created and think about it as having implications for other kinds of social movements invested in social change.

THIS IS FAT ACTIVISM

It is clear from the outset that, even within a small sample of people with shared social networks, fat activism is more than one thing and that the proxies I have identified from trying to find writing about fat activism are extremely limited. But more than that, the proxies are bad news for fat activists because they imply that activism is nonsensical, ineffectual, superficial and disorganised: a waste of time. One of the principal areas in which these claims are reproduced is in the idea that fat activism is not unified. Sara Ahmed proposes that this is a criticism often made by dominant cultures to suppress a plethora of minority culture opinions and that the drive to agree is one that sacrifices dissent, contradiction and difference, all of which are essential for social transformation.[1] In this section I am going to show that fat activism is a multifaceted affair, that unity is not as important as it might seem and suggest, as one participant explained: "There isn't a sort of uniform fat activist or activism" (Jamie).

When I asked people in the study "What is fat activism?" I was surprised by the responses. I thought they would know and have a pithy response at the ready. Some could not answer, others took much of the interview to answer it, others came back to it towards the end of the interview to reconsider their earlier responses. Of the people who answered, there were overlaps in what they said, but no two gave the same response, there was little consistency. Some people thought that it was a trick question. An assumption prevailed that people already knew and had agreed on a universal definition. People offered very precise definitions:

> I think of fat activism as being a response to the negative shit about fat. Challenging discourse, protesting stereotypes, countering fat hate, refusing to accept things, speaking truth to power, rejecting moral discourse concerning fatness, repudiating injustice. (Billy)

1 Sara Ahmed, "You Are Oppressing Us!" http://feministkilljoys.com/2015/02/15/you-are-oppressing-us/.

So I think fat activism is kind of like a way for fat people to engage in their own liberation, but larger than that, like address the ideas of what it means to have, to have a body, for it to be a commodity, and to be used against you, you know, and all sorts of things, for things like, for things like other people's moralisms or for commerce. (Liz)

But I found these too to be inadequate explanations for the breadth of activity that the participants described in the research. In the end, I identified five broad categories from the research data: political process activism; activist communities; fat activism as cultural work; micro fat activism and ambiguous fat activism. Fat activism is the stuff that people generally recognise as activism, but it is also the relationships between the people doing activism, it is the cultural work they produce, it can be very small moments that happen within or beyond community and it can be plain weird or quite horrible. These represent only a tiny fraction of the activities that could be thought of as fat activism because, as I show, fat activist methods can be anything, so they hint of unlimited possibilities. I should add that what people described as fat activism here very much represents the interests of the sample and what they considered valuable or relevant to the conversation so, for example, there is little about fatshion, Fat Studies and BBW cultures, all of which are major sites for fat activism in the West. The categories I have proposed are not mutually exclusive, instead the boundaries between them are permeable, and fat activist border crossings happen, perhaps inspired by life changes and ageing. Leora demonstrated this:

Um, I would say my fat activism has really run the gamut for a lot of different areas of life for me, so I feel like it's been everything from having frank discussions with my nieces and my family, just as treating it as a normal thing, which is difficult work to do, on-going work, and I think that I did not, it took a long time to learn how to deal with that really, and raise it, to, I've done a lot of vandalism over the years. On International No Diet Day[2] I would say I've definitely broken some laws to be disruptive, and vandalised diet centres. (Leora)

POLITICAL PROCESS FAT ACTIVISM

Political process activism follows a theory of public engagement with power proposed by Jürgen Habermas in *The Structural Transformation of the Public Sphere* and is closely connected to Western democratic ideology.[3] Here, social change is engendered through collective influence and public debate using the tools and processes of state power, for example through rights and policy.[4] This is what most people that I spoke to during the course of this work thought of as activism.

Tools and processes includes things like working within legal frameworks, as with Sondra Solovay's account of creating anti-fat discrimination legislation in San Francisco; through consumer advocacy, as with the Council on Size and Weight Discrimination and Allegro Fortissimo; or they might manifest through more prosaic means, such as street protest, public debate or letter-writing.[5]

2 6 May.
3 Jürgen Habermas, *The Structural Transformation of the Public Sphere: An Inquiry into a Category of Bourgeois Society*, Translated by Thomas Burger and Frederick Lawrence (Cambridge: Polity Press, 1989).
4 Anna Kirkland, *Fat Rights: Dilemmas of Difference and Personhood* (New York: New York University Press, 2008); Yofi Tirosh, "The Right to Be Fat," *Yale Journal of Health Policy, Law and Ethics*, XII, no. 2 (2012): 266-335.
5 Sondra Solovay, *Tipping the Scales of Justice: Fighting Weight-Based Discrimination* (Amherst, NY: Prometheus Books, 2000); CSWD, "Council on Size and Weight Discrimination," http://www.cswd.org/; Allegro Fortissimo, "Allegro Fortissimo," http://www.allegrofortissimo.com/. See also The Association for the Health Enrichment of Larger People (AHELP) which operated 1991-1996, Carol A. Johnson, *Self-Esteem Comes in All Sizes: How to Be Happy and Healthy at Your Natural Weight* (Carlsbad, CA: Gürze Books, 2001) and the International Size Acceptance Association for more in the same vein. ISAA, "International Size Acceptance Association," http://www.size-acceptance.org/.

In April, 1976, I wrote a letter to the [local council]. My action resulted in the council's voting to remove the 'weight loss' label from a summer movement programme it was offering. Because of my letter, the council expressly endorsed the right of fat women to participate in movement/exercises classes without fear of ridicule or harassment. (Dana)

Political process fat activism takes place in specialist organisations and also makes strategic use of existing structures and institutions. Eve's sub-group, for example, exerts influence through its visibility, and uses the power of the larger organisation to leverage its interests:

I don't think of myself as getting much done as a lone voice so what I try to do is create little subcultures wherever I am, so for example the [national organisation], we created the Health At Every Size[6] Special Interest Group because you can create special interest groups, it's fantastic. So we got our HAES SIG and we show up there at all the conferences with some sort of programming, we show up at other conferences with programming, we are on the main listserv for the [national organisation], which is a really

6 Health At Every Size (HAES) is a health paradigm that does not advocate remedial weight management. HAES practitioners Jon Robison and Linda Bacon outline three clear tenets: self-acceptance, joyful movement and intuitive eating. Jon Robison, "Health at Every Size: Toward a New Paradigm of Weight and Health," *Medscape General Medicine* 7, no. 3 (2005): 13; Jon Robison et al, "Health at Every Size: A Compassionate, Effective Approach for Helping Individuals with Weight-Related Concerns—Part I," *American Association of Occupational Health Nurses Journal* 55, no. 4 (2007): 143-50; Bacon, *Health at Every Size: The Surprising Truth About Your Weight*. Sometimes social justice or fat activism is included within the model but this cannot be assumed. Jacqueline Rochelle Gingras, *Longing for Recognition: The Joys, Complexities, and Contradictions of Practicing Dietetics* (York: Raw Nerve, 2009); Lucy Aphramor et al, "Critical Dietetics: A Declaration," *Practice*, no. 48 (2009): 2. In practice HAES is interpreted in multiple and apparently contradictory ways by health professionals working within traditional weight management models. Gail Marchessault et al, "Canadian Dietitians' Understanding of Non-Dieting Approaches in Weight Management," *Canadian Journal of Dietetic Practice and Research*, 68, no. 2 (2007): 67-72.

cool thing and actually there's a lot of discussion about clinical
stuff and social forces and political things and all sorts of things,
and it's a global community so it's really great because it's not just
the US. And we're a big time presence there. (Eve)

Institutional and professionalised, such organisations produce forms
of activism within them, such as fundraising and administrative work.

I'm on the board. I help to work on [a particular programme], and
I'm the Secretary of the board right now, which is interesting, so
I try to keep, I try to keep a sense of momentum in the stuff that
we're doing, I remind all of us, you know, of our different deadlines
and projects that we're working on. (Paz)

The mobilisation of people is important in political process fat activism
because it seeks mass influence, this is not something that can be
undertaken alone. Daniah lists the outreach projects that are central to
their activism:

Um, we've done, I've done workshops in so many different kinds
of spaces: schools, community events, LadyFests, queer events,
rush weeks, oh my god, like mostly for young, like, university
age, high school age, and younger, I've done a lot of work with
young, like, high school age girls. We have a bunch of conferences
that exist in [the city] for queer high school students, and so it's
spaces like that, Women's Studies, I've gone to classrooms and
lectured, stuff like that. So I've done workshops and I've done
lectures. (Daniah)

Public speaking forms a large part of this activism, and engaging with
various media is regarded as especially important because it reaches
large audiences. Impi expresses the difficulties of performing activism
in this context, she says of a colleague and herself:

> We have been both very active in the media, in that sense we have given those, sometimes those horrible statements to journalists who are clearly just basically idiots who don't really know what they're talking about or writing about but just trying to get your message across. If they want to know something about this, I try to say something positive in this horrible magazine! (Impi)

Political process fat activism is appealing because it offers a set of distinctly defined interests, aims and objectives founded on a sense of common purpose and oriented towards a progressive future. In using the tools and processes of the dominant culture, political process fat activism has a good chance of being recognisable and intelligible by that culture, ensuring its prominence, presence and legitimacy within a public sphere. Its rationale is to influence rather than re-order. It is no wonder that this form of activism has become the standard, it is almost generic.

But there are drawbacks. Not everybody has access and I will say much more about this in a later chapter. Although he refined his argument in later works, Habermas initially proposed that the idealised public sphere is built on a principle of universal access, of civilised debate. Nancy Fraser points out that this is naïve and that social inequality prevents people from participating and reproduces the usual power systems.[7] Furthermore, only certain kinds of subjects and ideas are permissible within a public sphere, Fraser argues that this is gendered because women tend to be associated with the private, but it also implies that people who don't use the dominant culture's ways of speaking, such as debate, are similarly excluded. This suggests that the people who participate in political process fat activism are those who already have privilege and resources. Moreover, although this type of activism is largely respectable and law-abiding, public protest is frequently criminalised and marginal people's involvement becomes increasingly risky.[8]

7 Nancy Fraser, "Rethinking the Public Sphere: A Contribution to the Critique of Actually Existing Democracy," *Social Text* 25, no. 26 (1990): 56-80.
8 Michael Welch, *Flag Burning: Moral Panic and the Criminalisation of Protest* (New York: Walter de Gruyter, 2000); Jennifer Earl, "Political Repression: Iron Fists, Velvet

There is another kind of naivety at play within this approach to
fat activism. Political process activism entails the work of delayed
gratification and self-sacrifice for the long-term project of social change,
but this is not guaranteed. Even if you have access, dominant culture can
be exploitative. For example, Paul McAleer documents instances in which
weight loss corporations have appropriated fat activist concepts;[9] merely
knowing and recognising fat activism does not ensure that dominant
interests will play fair.[10]

Political process fat activism is founded on an idea of universal rights
and justice.

> Well, activism is about creating justice, right, it's about working
> to create a world where there is justice for fat people as well as
> everyone else. (Elliot)

Justice is an attempt to engender accountability, but it is also associated
with authoritarian judgment, punishment, and social control.[11] Given
this, it is worth asking whose voices become lost or excluded when
organisations operate through conformity, agreement, sameness and
compromise. Rights discourses are problematic for other reasons, as
Anne Mulhall notes, they presume a modernist progression from savage
primitivism to urban sophistication and can invoke troubling Western
imperialism and colonialism, such as the enforcing of rights on others

Gloves, and Diffuse Control," *Annual Review of Sociology* 37, no. 1 (2011): 261-84.

9 As with whitewashing, defined as a cover-up and used to develop concepts such
as greenwashing (using ecological claims to hide environmental misconduct) and
pinkwashing (using an idea of gay-friendliness to hide oppressive regimes), I propose
fatwashing as the appropriation of fat activist and HAES ideas by weight loss advocates
and businesses to obscure their real nature.

10 Paul McAleer, "Weight Watchers Co-Opts Our Language," http://www.bigfatblog.
com/weight-watchers-co-opts-our-language.

11 Angela Y. Davis, *Are Prisons Obsolete?* (New York: Seven Stories Press, 2003); Eric
A. Stanley and Nat Smith, *Captive Genders: Trans Embodiment and the Prison Industrial
Complex* (Edinburgh: AK Press, 2011).

who do not share the same values.[12] The linear construction of progress does not allow for the complications and messiness of human behaviour in social movements[13] where collective process is often hard won.[14]

Where fat activism is always relative to dominant discourse, rather than formulated as an activity in its own right, paradoxically it may also reproduce it because the dominant culture's views are always there and always being reproduced through resistance.[15] But an investment in dominant culture cannot be assumed. In *Fat & Proud* I argued that fat hatred is closely allied to power and that the work of eliminating fat hatred is tied to that of dismantling fatphobic institutions and systems where power impacts negatively on marginalised people.[16]

> So, like I guess I don't like the idea of fat activism like beginning and ending with a rights-based movement, like "We the fat people are oppressed and we want equal rights under this system," to everything because I feel like it's that same [sort] of thing when, how do I want to say, like performance goals are necessary because people are suffering right now, and I don't want that to be the end point, like I don't want, you know, fatties to just be on *Vogue* magazine, or whatever, I want it to be much more broad than that.
>
> Charlotte: The system is shit, it has to change.
>
> Exactly! Like not a piece of the pie, the pie is rotten, let's get rid of the pie, or something, so. (Louisa)

12 Anne Mulhall, "Camping up the Emerald Aisle: Queerness in Irish Popular Culture" in *Irish Postmodernisms and Popular Culture*, edited by Wanda Balzano et al, 210-19 (Basingstoke: Palgrave Macmillan, 2007).

13 For example complicity, or the ambiguous borderlands between oppressor and oppressed.

14 Delfina Vannucci and Richard Singer, *Come Hell or High Water: A Handbook on Collective Process Gone Awry* (Edinburgh: AK Press, 2010).

15 Diamond, "Thin Is the Feminist Issue."

16 Cooper, *Fat & Proud: The Politics of Size.*

Instead of seeking rights within a system that she sees as corrupt, Louisa speaks in favour of fat activism that is part of a bigger revolutionary political ideal, and which might be one of the tools that enables her to dismantle the status quo.

ACTIVIST COMMUNITIES

Community-building is a part of political process activism, because it mobilises people, but my research indicates that it is also activism in its own right because it enables fat people to develop social capital. This follows the work of sociologists interested in social movements, who turned their attention from how people organise, to how people relate to each other as activists.[17] Although activists might still be pursuing political process goals, everyday interaction between members of activist communities, and the work of community-building is also important because it enables people to share information and develop new identities and interests.[18]

Sociologists have expanded the concept of capital beyond the realm of economics.[19] Having capital is not just about having money. Capital as wealth can include other forms, including cultural capital (taste, knowledge, education, for example), and social capital (networks that can influence or support people). Building community, simply getting together, is a project of generating social capital, developing connections that enable people to exercise power, become agentic and visible, and be

17 Alain Touraine, "On the Frontier of Social Movements," *Current Sociology* 52, no. 4 (2004): 717-25.

18 Fraser, "Rethinking the Public Sphere: A Contribution to the Critique of Actually Existing Democracy"; Steve Valocchi, "Riding the Crest of a Protest Wave? Collective Action Frames in the Gay Liberation Movement, 1969-1973," *Mobilization: An International Quarterly* 4, no. 1 (1999): 59-73.

19 Pierre Bourdieu, *Distinction: A Social Critique of the Judgement of Taste* (Cambridge, MA: Harvard University Press, 1984); Bourdieu, "The Forms of Capital"; Bev Skeggs, *Formations of Class & Gender* (London: SAGE, 1997).

legitimised.[20] Through community, fat activists perform the alchemical work of converting abjection into asset.[21] This is often gendered and embodied work.[22]

Though a central concept, community was rarely defined by the people I interviewed for this research, people took it for granted. Reese explained its significance:

> It's a network of people who share a common belief system, who do it lovingly. You know, it's people who you know will show up if you throw something, who will help you, like, spread the word. It's friendship, or acquaintanceship, or allies, I guess. I don't-, defining community, it's a place to go, you know, like whether it's like, like NOLOSE is a community, these people are banded together under this particular umbrella and certainly it feels safer to be with them than not. And also not, it brings up a lot of stuff for a lot of people, it's complicated but so's family, right? So, it's extended family, I guess. (Reese)

20 The London Fat Women's Group, The Weigh In, Fat Positivity Belgium, Fat Positive London are examples of this kind of community-building group, loosely-organised spaces where people might meet online and offline. Club nights such as Rebel Cupcake in Brooklyn and Dancing On My Own in London also produce fat community.
21 See these examples of community-based knowledge and skill-sharing: Nancy Barron's account of fat activist support groups; Lynn McAfee and Jean Soncrant's collaborative manual, which explains how fat people might negotiate restrictive airline travel; McAfee and Miriam Berg's outline of the basic skills required for advocating for rights for fat people, and for making complaints; and my guide for fat cyclists documents my own cycling experience with the aim of encouraging others to follow suit. Nancy Barron et al, "Fat Group: A Snap-Launched Self-Help Group for Overweight Women," *Human Organization,* 43, no. 1 (1984): 44-49; Nancy Barron and B.H. Lear, "Ample Opportunity for Fat Women," *Women and Therapy* 8 (1989): 79-82; Jean Soncrant and Lynn McAfee, "Airline Tips for Large Passengers," *Healthy Weight Journal* 15, no. 4 (2001): 63; Lynn McAfee and Miriam Berg, "Advocacy" in *Weight Bias: Nature, Consequences and Remedies,* edited by Kelly Brownell et al, 285-93 (New York: The Guilford Press, 2005); Charlotte Cooper, "How to Ride a Bike: A Guide for Fat Cyclists," http://charlottecooper. net/publishing/digital/how-to-ride-a-bike-a-guide-for-fat-cyclists-02-05/.
22 Bev Skeggs, *Class, Self, Culture* (London: Routledge, 2004).

Eve spelled out what community-building might look like:

> Well, the other part of the activism I guess is all the [organisational]
> infrastructure-building, community-building, [online
> messageboards], showing up, providing content, providing ways
> of talking about things, thinking about things, I guess I feel like
> I'm building ideas, and that's a lot of my activism is the building
> of ideas, to the extent that they have legs, they go out into the
> world and people mess with them and do whatever with them,
> and I'm just thrilled that that's going to be a legacy of mine, that
> I feel that that's what I love myself and the power of ideas in my
> life has been profound, and so I want to just carry that on, pass it
> on. I guess that's it. (Eve)

Community-building is what happens behind the scenes in other forms
of activism, but Kris pointed out that this hidden work is as important as
that which happens in front of the curtain. She described her participation
in a group which used street theatre and performance as its more public
face of fat activism at the turn of the millennium:

> And so we would do a performance maybe once a year, maybe twice
> a year, maybe even up to six times a year, but we would meet weekly
> almost throughout the whole year and those meetings were really,
> you know, now I wasn't really thinking about it at the time but in
> retrospect I can see that they were definitely consciousness-raising
> sessions. They were ways for us to connect and feel like we weren't
> alone, and create community, and share our experiences, and then
> articulate our experiences from being these sort of isolated and
> depressing moments into, not just a liberatory but kind of, I don't
> know, a way of thinking it through a group of people. Changing
> that experience in a way by coming together. (Kris)

The work of inviting people to participate in a discussion, to recognise
themselves as part of a community, can have powerful effects. Given the

lifelong isolation that many fat people have felt, being part of a community of people with shared values is psychologically important in claiming a strong self-identity, relinquishing loneliness, and finding people with whom to share experiences. This is reiterated in the following exchange:

> Charlotte: It is fabulous. When you encounter a proud freak or a bunch of proud freaks it is fucking fabulous.

> Yes and it makes me feel like I've found the people that I want to hang out with, and to me that's really it. (Kris)

Verity described how encountering community was crucial in her own identity development. She recalled the emotional intensity of her first encounter with community-building, at a reading by Judith Stein in the basement of New Words, a feminist book shop in Cambridge, Massachusetts:

> I think I've written about this, that Judy Freespirit and somebody else I didn't know well, but she was talked of in that way, and she was a writer, and the first time I heard her read it was the first time I'd heard like any lesbian feminist read, it was a fat woman, so it was in the basement of [unclear] so it was consciously fat women, and I sat in the back sobbing the whole time. Sobbing! Sobbing! Because she had named this opening for me. Talk about yeah, like "I can make the space so that you can walk through," I mean Judith made that space for me, she did. And so then, walking through it, I could say all these different things about "Well, I'm a writer and an activist" but it's the same thing, in some ways it is. I couldn't have even, I mean I was trying, but I couldn't have got there in the form that I did without that. (Verity)

In using community to generate capital, it helps to have pre-existing access to capital. Those without it may founder, as shown by the number of fat activist community groups that have failed to take off, of which more later. Elliott typifies this in her account of inviting people she encountered in her community to form a collective to produce a tangible object, a zine, in San Francisco the early 1990s. In her account she made indirect reference to cultural resources already available to her: zine-making and queer community, a Dyke March, the capital and skills required to make and distribute flyers, for example.

> Another thing I didn't say was that it wasn't just a group of people who knew each other, it started with a couple of people who knew each other, like five of us maybe, and then we started, it wasn't just at the Dyke March, we started going around and any time we would see a fat, queer, dykey, whatever person, um, we would invite them to come and be part of our group. I invited people I had never met, if I saw work they were doing that seemed really good, I saw my friend doing some performance art at [college], and I just walked up to her, I had never met her before, and I was like: "Do you want to be part of our zine for fat dykes?" [laughter]. And so there was a lot of reaching out to people, you know, er, it's like we really wanted to include the community, that was my personal mission, shared to varying degrees by different people.
>
> Charlotte: Right. So it emboldened you to do that?
>
> Yes! It really did. It was like: "Oh, I have this ruse for making a connection with you, and flirting with you," and all that, yeah! Yeah. (Elliot)

The capital intrinsic to this exchange is relatively modest, yet is cultivated to produce wide-ranging effects, there is a snowball effect. The flyers mentioned by Elliott were part of what generated submissions and volunteers who eventually produced the zine, as well as a readership. The zine not only helped reflect diverse fat perspectives within a queer subculture, but created a subculture and constituency of its own: "fat dykes." This had a big impact on people. Hannah was one of the fat dykes who encountered the zine produced by the collective later on, she recalls:

> So I took a Queer Studies class or something, I don't know that I was exposed to anything all that fascinating but while I was in the class, it was in this co-op at my school that I didn't normally go to and I was just like searching around in the bin and I found a copy of *FaT GiRL* that someone had just left around. I read it and my mind was just completely blown. I was like "I know what to do!" I was just so excited, I was like "WOW!" I think I was kind of turned off by the whole thing at first, I think I was like "Fuck! Oh my god! Ew!" but then I took it home and I was really like: "Oh my god, these people are wonderful, they're like the most wonderful people I have ever seen in my life. THESE ARE THE PEOPLE!" So I went from being horrified to being "Oh I'm so glad that there's people like that out there," to being "I'm moving to San Francisco and becoming a fat activist in a day and a half" [laughter]. (Hannah)

It is remarkable that an object as transient as an extinct collectively-produced zine about fat dykes, started through a campaign of flyering, flirting and word of mouth, should have such a far reach over time and place. In London I was given a flyer for *FaT GiRL* by a friend in 1993, I then sent off for a copy, had work published in it over the following years, visited the collective in San Francisco in 1996, made long-standing friendships, and continue to feel a deep connection to the project. I will say more about fat feminist travels later on.

Reese is astute in recognising that negotiating community can be complicated and uncomfortable. Community is an idea of something shared that reveals a great many divisions between community members.[23] People are generally members of different communities, some of which overlap and some of which are in conflict with each other.

23 Elana Dykewomon, "Lesbian Quarters," *Journal of Lesbian Studies* 9, no. 1-2 (2005): 31-43.

Here, community is networks where there are shared interests as well as differences, where there is potential for offering and accessing support. Hannah clarified this:

> And so I think for me [fat activism] just means this simple act of allowing yourself to be a valid person and taking other people with you when possible. (Hannah)

It would be a mistake to approach fat community only as spaces that are helpful, compassionate or encouraging; there may be in- and out-group tensions and political differences.[24] Marìa points to stresses that arose between different values in Bay Area fat feminist communities of the 1980s and 1990s, one a renunciation and the other a celebration.

> There was also a very clear anti-dieting kind of rhetoric that was part of it, that we will not participate in this act which is dangerous to us. So it was much more about, I think, at the time, it was much more about, "We are not going to do these injurious things, we will not participate and collude in our own destruction." And then there was a group that was more about "Fat is great!" you know, "Fat is beautiful," and sort of really being involved in terms of a Fat Pride kind of movement, and that was a big part of it. (Marìa)

Despite the friendly, welcoming rhetoric and public face of fat activist communities, some parts of the movement have a problem with bullying and bystanding.[25] It can be hard to keep going and difficult for people to show up. This suggests that organisations are not necessarily the founts of shared ethics and collective agreement that they are assumed to be in the literature of fat activism and that they contain a broad range of ideologies.

I have argued that community-building is activism, but this is a

---

24 Colls, "Big Girls Having Fun: Reflections on a 'Fat Accepting Space'"; Maya Maor, "The Body That Does Not Diminish Itself: Fat Acceptance in Israel's Lesbian Queer Communities," *Journal of Lesbian Studies* 16, no. 2 (2012): 177-98.

25 Cooper and Murray, "Fat Activist Community: A Conversation Piece."

contested claim. Liat recalled the community of fat lesbian feminist activists she was part of, a community that was both a political and social group. She implied that the social aspect of the group emerged after the politics were somehow attained or completed, suggesting that there was a clear distinction between their political activism and social activities.

> And there was a social life here with other fat women for a long time, I would say right through the '80s. You know, there were parties and there were people hooking up or whatever, there was a bunch of people who were all dating each other, or not dating each other, so that was always amusing. And you know there was just sort of more of a social scene, people would all go to a bar the same night and dance, or, you know, different things like that. But, you know, wasn't, there wasn't as much political activity, because it was like; "Ok so we have the politics, now we can have some fun." You know. (Liat)

Liat regards the social spaces as extraneous to the political work of fat activism. But this group were still doing fat activism through their relationships and in the social spaces they created together, even during their time off. To recognise oneself and others, to commit to a relationship, is a political act in a context where one's humanity is repeatedly diminished in the wider culture. I would maintain that such relationships could be understood as gestures of defiance, perhaps, or acts of survival, they are not secondary to the real work of activism, they are a central part of that work.

Furthermore, it is false to assume that there is a divide between doing activism and being within a community of activists. Fat activist community contests the distinctions between public and private, political and social, friend and comrade. For example, Sarah was part of a performance group in the Bay Area that was established in the early 1980s, membership changed over its lifespan but the group met "every Sunday, every Sunday with rare exceptions, for about 12 years." Fat activism here is not only in the performances the group produced together, but also in the commitment to meeting for such a long period, in being present for one another, in creating a collective space in which to explore what it is to be fat. Here fat activism is about witnessing each other rather than taking cues from dominant culture. Community-building enables fat activists to understand the conditions of our lives and to set agendas for change.

FAT ACTIVISM AS CULTURAL WORK

Creative and cultural expression forms a substantial part of fat activism.[26] Cultural work refers to the act of making things: art, objects, events, still and moving images, digital artefacts, texts, spaces, places and so on. Cultural production in fat activism encompasses art and photography that makes fat embodiment and fat activist community visible.[27] This cultural work includes the actions of fat activists as cultural critics.[28]

26 Leanne Cusitar et al eds, *The Fat Issue*. Edited by Caroline Sin, Shauna Lancit and Jessica Ticktin Vol. 67, Fireweed. (Toronto: Fireweed, 1999).

27 Anonymous, "Rachael Field's Paintings," *Spare Rib* no. 234 (1992): 21; Cath Jackson and Rachael Field, "Broadening Out," *Trouble & Strife* no. 23 (1992): 18-23; Laurie Toby Edison and Debbie Notkin, *Women En Large: Images of Fat Nudes*. 1st ed (San Francisco, CA: Books in Focus, 1994); Leonard Nimoy, *The Full Body Project: Photographs by Leonard Nimoy* (Minneapolis: Consortium, 2007); Substantia Jones, "The Adipositivity Project," http://www.adipositivity.com/; Allyson Mitchell, *Ladies Sasquatch* (Hamilton, Ontario: McMaster Museum of Art, 2009); Lauren Gurrieri, "Stocky Bodies: Fat Visual Activism," *Fat Studies: An Interdisciplinary Journal of Body Weight and Society* 2, no. 2 (2013): 197-209; Majida Kargbo, "Toward a New Relationality: Digital Photography, Shame, and the Fat Subject," *Fat Studies: An Interdisciplinary Journal of Body Weight and Society* 2, no. 2 (2013): 160-72. See also how art and community-building share common ground, such as the Fat Friday gatherings at the Vida Gallery in San Francisco in 1982, a series of poetry readings, performances, music, theatre and visual art.

28 See for example Le'a Kent, "Fighting Abjection: Representing Fat Women" in *Bodies out of Bounds: Fatness and Transgression*, edited by Jana Evans Braziel and Kathleen LeBesco, 130-50 (Los Angeles: University of California Press, 2001); Stefanie Snider, "Revisioning Fat Lesbian Subjects in Contemporary Lesbian Periodicals," *Journal of Lesbian Studies* 14, no. 2 (2010): 174-84; Jennifer-Scott Mobley, "Tennessee Williams' Ravenous Women: Fat Behavior Onstage," *Fat Studies: An Interdisciplinary Journal of Body Weight and Society* 1, no. 1 (2012): 75-90; Jennifer L. Graves and Samantha Kwan, "Is There Really 'More to Love'?: Gender, Body, and Relationship Scripts in

There are networks of fat activist cultural workers and cultural work is produced by communities, individually, or both, as Dana illustrated:

From 1973 through 1977, I contributed my essays and poetry to *Sister!* (a Los Angeles Feminist newspaper) [...] I also wrote several fat positive articles for *The Venice Beachhead* (a local alternative newspaper) during these years. I wrote *The Venice Beachhead* articles and the articles in *Sister!* independent of being in The Fat Underground, although I was supported and encouraged by the other fat activists. (Dana)

Like community-building, cultural work is activism that generates capital and socially transforms fat. Because it is interpretable and unfixed, it offers new possibilities for imagining fat, the first step towards creating change. There are sceptics who argue that this transformation has limited material benefits.[29] I disagree with this position and hope to demonstrate below that making culture has rich potential for social change. I will discuss some of the methods that fat activists use to create culture below but there is not room to address a comprehensive range of activities because these are extremely varied.

Romance-Based Reality Television," *Fat Studies: An Interdisciplinary Journal of Body Weight and Society* 1, no. 1 (2012): 47-60; Joyce L. Huff, "'Fattening' Literary History," *Fat Studies: An Interdisciplinary Journal of Body Weight and Society* 2, no. 1 (2013): 30-44; Johnanna J. Ganz, "'The Bigger, the Better': Challenges in Portraying a Positive Fat Character in Weeds," *Fat Studies: An Interdisciplinary Journal of Body Weight and Society*, 1, no. 2 (2012): 208-21; LeRhonda S. Manigault-Bryant, "Fat Spirit: Obesity, Religion, and Sapphmammibel in Contemporary Black Film," *Fat Studies: An Interdisciplinary Journal of Body Weight and Society* 2, no. 1 (2013): 56-69; Peter C. Kunze, "Send in the Clowns: Extraordinary Male Protagonists in Contemporary American Fiction," *Fat Studies: An Interdisciplinary Journal of Body Weight and Society* 2, no. 1 (2013): 17-29; Jackie Wykes, "'I Saw a Knock-Out': Fatness, (in)Visibility, and Desire in Shallow Hall," *Somatechnics* 2, no. 1 (2012): 60-79; Caroline Narby and Katherine Phelps, "As Big as a House: Representations of the Extremely Fat Woman and the Home," *Fat Studies: An Interdisciplinary Journal of Body Weight and Society* 2, no. 2 (2013): 147-59; Helen Hester and Caroline Walters, *Fat Sex: New Directions in Theory and Activism* (Farnham: Ashgate, 2015).
29 Murray, *The 'Fat' Female Body*.

Existing cultural forms

According to my research, fat activists use whatever resources available to them in order to produce culture. Daniah made creative use of graffiti, for example:

> So the [group] started off as picking up Sharpies and writing [our name] and other words pertaining to fat and queers all over [the city] in bathrooms in queer spaces and non-queer spaces, and it was basically about making the word visible, Fat, making fat visible, the word. And wondering, like thinking about what would happen when people are taking a dump or taking a piss and they're looking at these words, [our name], what are they thinking about, what is the jog for their brain? (Daniah)

New accessible online technologies have enabled other fat activists to develop cultural practice and build community. Rosa, a photographer, used her blog to expand notions of the "aesthetic validity" of fat with carefully constructed collaborative photographs of the fat people, mostly women, she met in her everyday life. She called this "photoactivism".

> Many of these people have never gotten naked in front of another person that they're not sexual with, it's a totally new experience, and I think that for anyone would be exhilarating, and then to see their naked body on the internet. It can be exhilarating, but when you factor in that we have bodies that society wants us to be ashamed of, wants us to hide under tent dresses, and teaches us that we should not have any pride and should not expect someone else to look at it as a thing of beauty, or even just to look at it, that adds a whole other level of power to it. (Rosa)

Other examples of fat activist cultural work that emerged through my research included sculpture, film, leading religious services, authoring books, and singing.[30] Susan Stinson argues that fiction is crucial for fat activists because it can deepen fat activist empathy, imagination and possibility.[31] This can be seen in the fat characters of her own novels.[32] Similarly complex representations of fat people can be found in other works of fiction and poetry by writers with roots in fat activism.[33] Zines also contribute to the fat activist artistic and literary canon.[34]

30 For a more in-depth discussion of how some contemporary fat activists use visual cultures read Stefanie Snider's paper on the topic. Stefanie Snider, "Fatness and Visual Culture: A Brief Look at Some Contemporary Projects," *Fat Studies: An Interdisciplinary Journal of Body Weight and Society* 1, no. 1 (2012): 13-31.

31 Susan Stinson, "Fat Girls Need Fiction" in *The Fat Studies Reader*, edited by Esther Rothblum and Sondra Solovay, 231-34 (New York: New York University Press, 2009).

32 Susan Stinson, *Fat Girl Dances with Rocks* (New York: Spinsters Ink, 1994); Susan Stinson, *Martha Moody* (London: The Women's Press, 1996); Susan Stinson, *Venus of Chalk* (Ann Arbor, MI: Firebrand Books, 2004).

33 Grace Nichols, *The Fat Black Woman's Poems* (London: Virago, 1984); Christine Donald, *The Fat Woman Measures Up* (Charlottetown, P.E.I: Ragweed, 1986); Susan Koppelman, ed. *The Strange History of Suzanne Lafleshe (and Other Stories of Women and Fatness)* (New York: The Feminist Press at the City University of New York, 2003); Kathy Barron et al, *Fat Poets Speak: Voices of the Fat Poets Society*, edited by Frannie Zellman (Nashville TN: Pearlsong Press, 2009); Sarai Walker, *Dietland* (New York: Houghton Mifflin, 2015).

34 Some examples: Hanne Blank, *Zaftig! Sex for the Well Rounded [Zine]* (Boston MA: Zaftig! Productions, 1999); Homo Ludenz, *At the Jungle Gym* (Berlin: Homo Ludenz, n.d. Zine); Rachel Kacenjar, *Free for Chubbies: A Fatshionista's Mini Guide to Repurposing and Reshaping Clothing [Zine]* (Cleveland, OH2008. zine); Nomy Lamm, *I'm So Fucking Beautiful [Zine]* (Olympia, WA1994. zine); FaT GiRL Collective, *Fat Girl* (San Francisco, CA: FaT GiRL, 1994); Taueret and Bunny, *Glutton for Fatshion [Zine]* (New York2009. zine; Taueret and Bunny, *Glutton for Fatshion #2 [Zine]* (Vol. 2, New York2010. zine); Max Airborne and Cherry Midnight, *Size Queen* (Oakland, CA: Size Queen, 2005); M@CE, *Venus Envy [Zine]* (Venus Envy. Terre Haute, IN1993. zine); V Vale, "Fat Girl," in *Zines! Volume One: Incendiary Interviews with Independent Publishers*, edited by V. Vale, 130-49 (San Francisco: Re/Search Publications, 1999); Krissy Durden, *Figure 8 [Zine]* (Portland, OR: Ponyboy Press, 2001-2009. Zine; Anonymous, *Hunger Strike [Zine]*, In the Spirit of Emma (London n.d. zine); Heather McCormack, "Fat Activism and Body Positivity: Zines for Transforming the Status Quo," *Library Journal*, http://reviews.libraryjournal.com/2012/03/collection-development/zines/fat-activism-and-body-positivity-zines-for-transforming-the-status-quo/; Charlotte Cooper, "A Queer and Trans Fat Activist Timeline - Zine Download," http://charlottecooper.net/b/oral-history/a-queer-and-trans-fat-activist-timeline/; Shannon Lee, *Fatty Fashions [Zine]*. 2006; Charlotte Cooper et al, "Big Bums [Zine]" (London, 2008); Kirsty Fife, "Make It Work: A Diy Fatshion Zine," Leeds, 2012; Kirsty Fife, "Make It Work #2," n.d;

Performance is particularly important within fat activist culture as a means of developing capital because of the immediacy of fat embodiment, its use as a reflection of fat experience, and its audiences as gatherings of fat community.[35] Within fat activist performance, dance, burlesque and drag create popular, playful experimental spaces.[36] In the UK, queer arts traditions and live art overlap in the production of fat activist performance spaces.[37] Andrea Elizabeth Shaw points out that performance is an area in which fat black women thrive.[38] As I write this, fat activism and dance are enjoying renewed visibility thanks to productions such as *SWAGGA* by Project O, and *Nothing to Lose* by Force Majeure[39] but fat activist dance has a long history. Sarah recalled the shift that occurred in her upon attending *We Dance*, Deb Burgard's innovative dance classes for fat women in the Bay Area in the late 1980s:

> And so Deb's class was such a joy. But I started it in these like baggy clothes and all, and we had mirrors, and I wouldn't look at myself,

Holly Casio, "Joining the Dots: A Queer Fat Positive Perzine About Pcos," 2012; Kirsty Fife, "I Love Myself: A Self Care Zine," n.d; Kirsty Fife, "Hard Femme," 2013-2015. See also poetry chapbooks Susan Stinson, *Belly Songs: In Celebration of Fat Women* (Northampton, MA: Susan Stinson, 1993, Chap Book); Judy Freespirit, *A Slim Volume of Fat Poems* (Oakland CA: Judy Freespirit, 1996).

35 Mitchell, "Pissed Off"; Vikki Chalklin, "All Hail the Fierce Fat Femmes" in *Fat Sex: New Directions in Theory and Activism*, edited by Helen Hester and Caroline Walters, 104-19 (Farnham: Ashgate, 2015).

36 Heather McAllister, "Embodying Fat Liberation" in *The Fat Studies Reader*, edited by Esther Rothblum and Sondra Solovay, 305-10 (New York: New York University Press, 2009); D. Lacy Asbill, "'I'm Allowed to Be a Sexual Being': The Distinctive Social Conditions of the Fat Burlesque Stage" in *The Fat Studies Reader*, edited by Esther Rothblum and Sondra Solovay, 299-304 (New York: New York University Press, 2009); Jamie Ratliffe, "Drawing on Burlesque: Excessive Display and Fat Desire in the Work of Cristina Vela," *Fat Studies: An Interdisciplinary Journal of Body Weight and Society* 2, no. 2 (2013): 118-31.

37 See the work of Katy Baird, Mathilda Gregory, Holestar, Amy Lamé, Le Gâteau Chocolat, Kayleigh O'Keefe, Scottee and Selina Thompson, for example.

38 Shaw, *The Embodiment of Disobedience: Fat Black Women's Unruly Political Bodies*.

39 Cooper, C. "I Am a Fat Dancer, but I Am Not Your Inspiration Porn," *OpenDemocracy*, https://www.opendemocracy.net/transformation/charlotte-cooper/i-am-fat-dancer-but-i-am-not-your-inspiration-porn.

I'd just stare at Debbie besides trying to make sure I was doing the steps right and having fun. But from that, little by little I started watching other people in the class, and I, there started to be this shift in my vision, and I was like noticing how beautiful there were parts of, like how their cha-cha moved as my mother would say, their arms would wiggle, and their bellies and their thighs and everything, and just seeing the joy that they were having, and the fun that they were having. And one day it just happened and I slipped into view too, and I saw that I was like, my face looked like theirs, the joy of movement. (Sarah)

Some performers complicate the ways that cultural capital is produced by performing with fat bodies. Kris makes exposing her fat body part of her performance:

I do performance now and again, a few times a year and I tend to show a lot of my body when I do that, by either wearing outrageously tight outfits or, you know, a t-shirt that is too small and rides up and I don't pull it down. (Kris)

But for Benjamin displaying his body onstage raises questions about the responsibility of performing fatness.

Very few people have seen a body like mine undressed and it's like, you know, a naked, gender-variant, large- and, I, so I just know that I, I don't wanna do that lightly. And so I just like don't want to make that choice by default. So I just like really, I haven't been like getting undressed as often, and I am just kind of like I think of my body with a lot of responsibility in there too. [...]And in some ways that's just taking care of my audience, I think it's also about artistry. I have something that I can get a reaction with, it's on me, I don't necessarily, I want to be careful with that. [...] I think that people definitely see my fat before they see anything else. (Benjamin)

Kris and Benjamin's performance choices are marked by their different backgrounds, including gender and ethnicity. But their decisions to show or not to show are informed by the idea that fat bodies are valuable and that knowledge generated by embodiment is also precious. Nevertheless, disclosing and transmitting that knowledge to audiences entails caution and, perhaps, responsibility.[40]

Other forms of fat activist cultural expression emerge from sex as an available and pre-existing resource. Sarah remembered going to a play party, a social space for public sex, that was organised by a younger generation of queer fat activists in the early 1990s:

> I remember [my girlfriend] and I went to, it was a *FaT GiRL* fundraiser, it was a big play party at this, I don't remember where, it was in San Francisco someplace, and that was a lot of fun but it was, you know, not my Mama's activism! (Sarah)

Fat activist culture-making here takes the form of exposure to and participation in forbidden forms of fat embodiment mediated through desire. This happens in other fat and queer sexualised spaces, such as porn and sex work. It also happens through projects like *The Den of Desire*, a free volunteer brothel that was organised by fat activists at a national queer conference in the US in 2010 and 2011 so that all who wanted to could assert a basic right to consensual sexual expression with someone else.[41] The play party, or sex party, is already

40 Benjamin's reflections on the politics of disclosing his body in public echo a recent campaign in which advice was circulated to help prevent fat people's pictures being used to market fatphobia or weight loss without the model's consent. Charlotte Cooper, "Headless Fatties, the Visual Cliché That Will Not Die" in *Obesity Timebomb*, 2012, http://obesitytimebomb.blogspot.co.uk/2012/01/headless-fatties-visual-cliche-that.html.

41 Christine and Deva, *Heavy Sm: Fat Brats Speak Out*, edited by Fish San Francisco: Brat Attack: The Zine for Leatherdykes and Other Bad Girls [zine], 1991; Drew Campbell, "Confessions of a Fat Sex Worker" in *Whores and Other Feminists*, edited by Jill Nagle, 189-90 (New York: Routledge, 1997); Kitty Stryker, "Fat Sex Works!" in *Hot & Heavy: Fierce Fat Girls on Life, Love & Fashion*, edited by Virgie Tovar (Berkeley, CA: Seal Press, 2012); April Flores, "Voluptuous Life" in *Hot & Heavy: Fierce Fat Girls*

a transgressive space but, when appropriated by "fat dykes and the women who want them"[42], it creates a unique time and place, which endures in community memory, where fat queer sexuality is central.[43]

New cultural forms

As well as developing and synthesising existing forms, fat activism has invented its own tactics to build community and cultural capital. Here I will briefly mention fat swims, fatshion and clothing swaps. These reflect the popularity and mainstreaming of alternative fat approaches to health and fashion.

Fat people cannot normally be tolerated in the states of undress required to swim, especially as a group, without being the target of unwanted attention. Fat swims are swimming sessions, usually held in accessible pools away from the view of outsiders, where fat people and their friends and loved ones can swim together and socialise around a pool without being harassed. Fat swims were first organised by lesbian fat activists in the San Francisco Bay Area in the early 1980s, the strategy has travelled to other places since then, and they are a feature of national gatherings in the US such as NAAFA and NOLOSE. Fat swims are

on Life, Lover & Fashion, edited by Virgie Tovar, 121-25 (Berkeley, CA: Seal Press, 2012); Hester and Walters, Fat Sex: New Directions in Theory and Activism.

42 FaT GiRL's maxim.

43 I would like to compare this instance of how fat activists talk about fat sexuality with that proposed by Ariane Prohaska, who creates a "a sexual deviance typology" of feeders (people who fetishise weight gain) she studied via online fora and characterises fat community spaces as "communal deviance". To me this typifies the problematic nature of an allegedly enlightened research gaze into fat and sexuality where community engagement is absent and fat people are reduced to pieces of data. Ariane Prohaska, "Help Me Get Fat! Feederism as Communal Deviance on the Internet," Deviant Behavior 35 (2014): 263–74. I would also like to refer readers to my own list of obesity researcher types, a tongue-in-cheek response to the obesity research obsession with typologies of fat people which, in my opinion, are reminiscent of the Victorian categorisation of sexuality to which Foucault refers in his classic work. Foucault, The History of Sexuality, Vol. 1; Charlotte Cooper, "The Six Types of Obesity Researcher," Obesity Timebomb, http://obesitytimebomb.blogspot.co.uk/2015/04/the-six-types-of-obesity-researcher.html.

heterotopic[44] because they create an alternative space in which being fat is normalised and can be enjoyed playfully and socially. Fat swims can be seen as part of a HAES strategy for activity that does not stigmatise weight, and swims are characterised by an atmosphere of well-being and socialising rather than training. Performance projects that incorporate synchronised swimming such as The Padded Lillies and Aquaporko are part of this tradition.[45]

There is evidence that, for some time, plus-size clothing retailers have used strategies familiar to fat activists to market their products, suggesting a close relationship between capitalism and some forms of activism.[46] More recently, fat activists have sought to explore and critique this relationship. *Fatshionista*, a LiveJournal online community, was originally intended as a place to discuss the politics, ethics and aesthetics of fat and fashion raised by the marketing of fat in the plus-size clothing industry.[47] The community generated a number of practises including outfit-blogging, where participants post an image of themselves in an outfit they like and invite comments from readers. In this way, fatshion encourages fat people's creative participation in spaces where they are usually excluded. I will say more about fatshion later on.

Clothing swaps were popularised by fat feminist activists in the US as a means of acquiring difficult-to-find affordable large-sized clothing and sharing garments as a community resource. The Fat Girl Flea Market refashioned this idea. The first Flea took place in New York in 2004 as a fundraiser for NOLOSE, it has continued sporadically since then

44 Heterotopias are places that disrupt normative concepts of space and time to create windows of possibility in which other ways of being that cannot normally be tolerated have opportunities to thrive. Michel Foucault and Jay Miskowiec, "Of Other Spaces," Architecture /Mouvement/ Continuité, http://foucault.info/documents/heteroTopia/foucault.heteroTopia.en.html; Judith Halberstam, *In a Queer Time & Place: Transgender Bodies, Subcultural Lives* (New York: New York University Press, 2005).

45 Shirley Sheffield, "Padded Lillies," http://paddedlilies.com/; Kelli Jean Drinkwater, "Aquaporko: The Documentary," http://aquaporkofilm.com/.

46 Pathé, *Plump and Lovely (Miss Fat and Beautiful Contest) [Video].* London: Pathé, 1962.

47 Amanda Piasecki, "Fatshionista," http://community.livejournal.com/fatshionista/.

and has inspired similar events elsewhere, including the 2010 Big Bum Jumble in the UK. Liz was instrumental in setting up the Flea, now called The Big Fat Flea:

> So the Flea grew over the years that we did it, we always do it at the Gay and Lesbian Centre, so there's a certain level of, like, you have to be willing to walk into the Lesbian and Gay Community Centre, but sometimes people's desire for inexpensive clothing trumps whatever–
>
> Charlotte: Their homophobia!
>
> Trumps their homophobia! Shopping trumps a lot of things! It really really does. It's a really powerful tool in, like, you don't think about it but you're not inviting people in to, say, support being queer, but there's a certain level of acceptance or support or at least tolerance or a lack of intolerance even in that moment, to, like, walk in that door and pay your $5 or whatever, and then rummage through an insane amount of clothing and walk out with your stuff, and then hopefully what people experience in the space of the Fat Girl Flea Market is an idea of community, is an idea of body, or people who are actively choosing to not engage in self-hate culture, not engage in dieting as a, whatever, self-punishing activity, and choose to do things differently. But you don't actually have to subscribe to it to participate, because our goal is to make as much money as we can so that people who want to be fat activists can participate and create community. But it definitely reaches, like, you know, I mean there're just like church ladies with four kids who come in and get 50 bags of clothes, and they're doing it because they have a particular need. So it makes me happy that we're creating a space in which multiple needs are met and it's not, it's not about dogma, it's about kind of the, you know, it's still the reality that there's a lack of accessible clothing out there. (Liz)

Not all clothes swaps take place in this way, some are small gatherings of people allied to social networks, but the Flea remains the biggest of these events. By capitalising on the mainstreaming of fat fashion, the Flea has become a popular and accessible event but it has not done so at the expense of its roots in queer community. Instead, it has created a cross-cultural space for community-building and the development of fat cultural capital in which people can find what they need and want without judgement, which supports a celebratory atmosphere, centred on an abundance of cheap recycled clothing.

MICRO FAT ACTIVISM

The fat activism I've described so far is at least recognisable as activism, whether or not it appears as such in the current body of literature. But micro fat activism is where my research starts to deviate from standard definitions of activism in Western scholarship.

Political process and the work of community and culture-building enables social movements to be theorised as largely collective endeavours. But organisations, even loose and informal groups, cannot meet their members' interests at all times. Fat activism has a wide repertoire of methods and strategies and, although the people in the sample reported engaging with fat activism of different types, their most numerous accounts by far were activities and interventions that I call micro fat activism.

Micro fat activism takes place in everyday spaces, is generally performed by one person, sometimes two, but rarely more, and happens in small, understated moments. Micro fat activism requires few material resources, and is not dependent on place, for example it is not necessarily an urban phenomenon. It is an activism that can engage people who might find other forms of activism inaccessible or exclusive. Micro fat activism does not rely on collective action, it can involve very small acts undertaken in isolation. This type of activism might be the only way in which people perform fat activism, or it might be carried out in conjunction with other forms. Where political process fat activism is built on a promise of delayed gratification, micro fat activism is immediate, there is no need to mobilise large numbers of people, or attract the attention of the great and the good, it can be undertaken now, in the moment. Such interventions represent the dynamic ways in which fat activists take fat activism into their own hands. Following this, the people I interviewed spoke of activities such as researching someone or something online, sending off for books, stealing office equipment from work to make flyers, surviving, buying things, exercising, learning, playing with one's identity. Micro fat activism is underscored by thought and intention, but it is not always public. It can involve choosing to eat something, for example, or making an accessible home for oneself, as described here by Marìa:

> Downstairs has one of those taller toilets too, it's kind of nice to have a house where you can make it fat friendly, with outdoor furniture that is fat friendly. I can sit on it and have room, and it's, you know, nice to be in a place where you feel comfortable. (Marìa)

This kind of fat activism is often conversational. Martha described the activism involved in speaking out or speaking back to fatphobic comments where she worked:

> So all that workplace conversation about food being bad. So I spent time trying to figure out what can I say where I don't want to engage, and I don't want to really come out as a radical fat activist, and I don't want to listen to this, and I don't need to slay the person for saying it, so what can I say? So that's where we started coming up with language like: "I don't think food is good or bad." (Martha)

This is the work of gently – or not so gently! – drawing people's attention to micro-oppression, but it also involves being visible to others in an unthreatening way and bringing fat consciousness to other conversations, for example in friendships. This could be seen as a form of identity politics. Calling-out is the act of identifying and refusing oppressive behaviour, often in the moment, by speaking about it in public and is often a strategy of exercising identity politics. It involves a personal act of speaking in order to assert collective responsibility, and it can be a challenging process. But calling-out should not be regarded as synonymous with micro fat activism, even though both are often responses to micro-aggressions, micro fat activism includes other strategies, of which calling-out is one example.

The quiet spaces of micro fat activism are overlooked in sociological grand narratives of social movements, but they are theorised more readily in feminist accounts that emphasise the value of lived experience.[48] This is evident in a long account from Martha, who described micro fat activism as personal development which led to an awakening:

> Somewhere in the, probably like '74 or '-5, I had already come out, so I was a lesbian, I was living in a group house, and I saw something about the Fat Liberator Publications, which might have been in *Lesbian Connection* magazine, I can't remember where I saw it, and I sent for it and I can't particularly remember why I sent for it except something about it grabbed me. And they came and I read 'em and I think there was a kind of an infiltration process and I was a feminist and I was a lesbian and I was an activist. I was working in women's healthcare at the time in a community-run health centre, and so to me it all came from there, and then I had a kind of an epiphany at an event, and I could tell you that pretty briefly, and then from that I said, well what happened was I used to sew and I made myself a pair of pants to wear to a concert, a lesbian concert, and they were just drawstring waist so they didn't pull me in at all, and wearing them I was so conscious that for the first time I wasn't wearing, like, jeans that sort of held on my stomach or anything that held me in, so throughout this whole

48 Nancy A. Naples and Karen Bojar, *Teaching Feminist Activism: Strategies from the Field* (New York: Routledge, 2002).

concert while I was listening to the music I was also thinking: "This is big, this thing of wearing these loose pants, and maybe they even make me look fatter," who knows, you know, but that was all in my mind, and I had good friends, they were good lesbian feminists, and I thought: "Not one of these women will really get what this is about. They would support me, they would be glad for me, they would do all those things and they wouldn't get it in themselves," because none of them were fat. So I did what seemed natural at that moment which was I organised a fat lesbian support group. And so, you know, I, that's not everybody-, I don't know, that's just what I did. So that, I think the first meeting was in 1978, it was in January and my friend Marcia remembers the date exactly, but I don't, I never remember quite if it was '78 or '79. But that was how it started. I wanted to have a place to talk about what it meant to be a fat woman wearing clothes that didn't pull me in, as just one example of the whole spectrum. (Martha)

It could be argued that micro fat activism is an activism of solipsistic individualism, but Martha's example is embedded in community. Micro fat activism could be understood as a form of minority influence, it acts as a method of opinion changing.[49] Deborah Martin et al. regard the small, everyday actions that are central to micro fat activism as the beginnings of community-building.[50] This supports Martha's experience in doing "what seemed natural" at the time and forming a support group. But whilst Martin and her co-authors envisage micro fat activism as a kind of pre-activism that inevitably leads to more traditional styles of activism, Sara O'Shaughnessy and Emily Huddart Kennedy regards it as valid in its own right because it represents actions that encourage, demonstrate or communicate an alternative way of being.[51] This suggests that imagining

49 Wendy Wood et al, "Minority Influence: A Meta-Analytic Review of Social Influence Processes," *Psychological Bulletin* 115, no. 3 (1994): 323-45.
50 Deborah G. Martin et al, "What Counts as Activism? The Role of Individuals in Creating Change," *Women's Studies Quarterly* 35, no. 3&4 (2007): 78-94.
51 Sara O'Shaughnessy and Emily Huddart Kennedy, "Relational Activism:

other possibilities and acting on them is a fundament of micro fat activism.

Micro fat activism is real activism in its own right because it has powerful effects. Activism that is very small may suffer for its invisibility but it is also more difficult to place under surveillance, to police, control and criminalise. It is similarly subversive because it is accessible. The immediacy of micro fat activism, particularly its quiet relational qualities and use of assertiveness strategies produces embodied esteem within its practitioners and supports them in creating liveable lives for themselves and others. In this way subtle personal and social transformations take place, as noted by Helen:

> I think the most immediate thing is to make living a life easier, like living, living fat, being fat, embodying fat, less abjected, less self-flagellating and self-loathing, and that's certainly been a kind of really obvious benefit of fat activism for me. (Helen)

Some study participants were very certain that micro fat activism is a legitimate type of fat activism. Verity recalled the influence of US radical lesbian feminism in the 1980s on her sense of self as a fat activist; here identity itself is activism:

> It was so related to grassroots lesbian feminism and the idea was: "Yes, you're an activist, of course you're an activist, we're all activists. If you take the, if you proudly claim the word 'fat' and walk through the world doing that, that's activism". (Verity)

Liat is also an older activist who shares a background in radical lesbian feminism with Verity. She was adamant of the validity of micro fat activism and placed it at the centre of her practice unapologetically:

Reimagining Women's Environmental Work as Cultural Change," *Canadian Journal of Sociology/Cahiers Canadiens de Sociologie* 35, no. 4 (2010): 551-72.

So I see the entire spectrum and I think that a lot of us are fat activists and we may not ever go to a rally again but we do things in our own communities or in our own lives too. (Liat)

Julia, who comes from a different background to Liat and Verity, recognised that there are many possible ways of being a fat activist. She observed this in the actions of a performer she admired:

Because it's like, Beth Ditto's a fat activist but I don't know whether she actually does any "organising." (Julia)

Positioning micro fat activism as activism is contentious, despite the strength of opinion in its favour. Many of the activists I interviewed for this project reproduced perceived divisions between primary and secondary activism. The work a fat activist might undertake to develop self-acceptance, for example, is distinguishable though related to the bigger work, as explained by Leora:

Even people who have a good relationship with their body have this regular, on-going work that they do to keep that up, and I feel that that's different to fat activism, in a way. But of course they're [Charlotte interrupts and then shuts up] but they're like siblings to me. (Leora)

Kris described a philosophical division between what she called formal and informal activism.

Well formal would have been more like organising a group of people to do something in a public way that had an explicit message. And informal is more day to day life through the connections that I make, talking about food, and bodies and health, but not necessarily doing it in a costume with a leaflet and stickers. (Kris)

Julia described boundary policing within her activist communities about what constitutes activism. Here it is more allied to political process activism using direct action tactics:

> It's policed quite a lot in [the German city where I live], possibly in the UK as well. I mean here an activist is more, you're considered an activist if you're more of the banner-holding variety, and that you have to be doing something specifically about changing, changing the administration of the world. (Julia)

Paz observed that micro fat activism gets lost where there are already diverse forms of action:

> I think that often a thing that happens with people who are in identity-focused movements and-, which is that a lot of the personal work in a lot of the personal liberation work that ties in to movements for change gets lost and doesn't get defined as part of it. [...] fat folks who are doing different things, they often don't see themselves as being activists when they do things like intervene, when they do things like take a moment to talk to somebody at their workplace or interrupt something. And I feel like a lot of activism is about those personal moments. (Paz)

By adopting a hierarchical understanding of activism, one that privileges certain forms over others, fat activists are stuck between what is commonly understood as activism, and what they actually do in the everyday. This is not surprising given the preponderance of political process activism as the definitive form, with all other interventions treated as poor relations. But Chris Bobel argues that people who do activism do not necessarily think of themselves as activists because they have a perfect standard of activism against which they measure themselves.[52] This is true of fat

---

52 Chris Bobel, "'I'm Not an Activist Though I've Done a Lot of It': Doing Activism, Being Activist and the 'Perfect Standard' in a Contemporary Movement," *Social*

activists who do fat activism but who do not recognise themselves as
activists because they think of fat activism as being something that is
produced by special people under special circumstances. Bobel states
that the perfect standard is unattainable and diminishes people and their
actions. Her findings suggest that it is false to categorise some forms of
activism as more legitimate than others. I hope that fat activists might
be reassured by her argument and also take heed of and encouragement
from hooks' and Ian Maxey's insistence that activists reclaim the quiet,
inclusive and broad work of emancipation as an everyday activity. In
doing so it is possible to address the multiplicity of sites of oppression
that saturate everyday life.[53] This too is activism.

AMBIGUOUS FAT ACTIVISM

During the process of analysing the research interviews for this project,
I became interested in the accounts people gave of fat activism that
didn't fit the previous categories. One example is fat activist pedagogy,
which spreads across the categories I have laid out into culture-making,
community-building, micro activism and political process work and
gives pause for thought about how payment affects activism.[54] There
were other forms of fat activism that intrigued me because they weren't
part of a political process model or concerned with building community
and culture. Sometimes they were related to micro fat activism but
they had a weirder quality to them. I started to think of this material as
ambiguous fat activism because its context, execution and effects were
not very straightforward.

Movement Studies 6, no. 2 (2007): 147-59.

53 bell hooks, *Outlaw Culture: Resisting Representations* (New York: Routledge, 1994);
Ian Maxey, "Beyond Boundaries? Activism, Academia, Reflexivity and Research," *Area*
31, no. 3 (1999): 199-208.

54 Julie Guthman, "Teaching the Politics of Obesity: Insights into Neoliberal Embodiment
and Contemporary Biopolitics," *Antipode: A Radical Journal of Geography* 41, no. 5
(2009): 1110-33; Erin Cameron, "Teaching Resources for Post-Secondary Educators
Who Challenge Dominant 'Obesity' Discourse," *Fat Studies: An Interdisciplinary Journal
of Body Weight and Society* 4, no. 2 (2015).

For example, odd moments arise where there is a clear division between what is and what is not fat activism. People within the study sample complained about how limited conceptualisations of fat activism created frustratingly narrow discourse, and resulted in their withdrawal from the movement, to a greater or lesser extent.

> And then there's some kind of fat activism, like we've talked about this, there's something going on right now called something like, I can't remember what it's called, revolution or something, a new year resolution? A new year revolution? They're sending out, I think to a really a large number of people or at least 100 people, little emails that are, you know, "love your body," very simplistic, and they feel very prescriptive and reductive, and I find them really... and for those I like "unclick" and don't support, and complain to my friend about them! (Verity)

Here the mass email is constructed as "fat activism" but Verity's critical appraisal and abandonment of it is not. Nevertheless, it could be perceived as activism even though Verity presents her ambivalence as part of the problem. However I believe her resistance to the emails could be seen as activism.

In this chapter I have given examples of activism that produce objects, moments and spaces, documentation, or which exists through relationships. Hannah proposed that this form of materiality matters within activism and that her preference was for activism that entails labour:

> Well, like, the doing, both the intense personal work and work in the world of manifesting whatever it is that you're trying to do, whether that's making change happen, or running a film festival, or surviving, writing a book, doing actual labour to... One of the reasons why I have such a hard time with the burlesque culture is because I'm like, "What work is involved with that?" I know there's work involved in taking off your clothes and the personal work, but where's the work? Show me the work! (Hannah)

Activism is labour but ambiguous fat activism does not necessarily produce the kind of materiality to which Hannah refers. It can also be activism that is not there, it has no presence, for example in the act of not doing something. This is not necessarily a provocation, I will talk about anti-social activism below, it is more like an absence. Liz pointed out that fat activists can be:

> People who are actively choosing to not engage in self-hate culture, not engage in dieting as a, whatever, self-punishing activity, and choosing to do things differently. (Liz)

Ambiguous fat activism can be immaterial in other ways, it can be the work of imagination, or fantasy, or the enjoyment in reading accounts of fat activism. Verity explained:

> I take the witnessing very seriously, like sort of, so I love to see things developing, I love to see the accounts on the internet, and that can be internationally, I mean I'm monolingual so for me it has to be in English, but to get glimpses of what things are going on in other places, I get reports back about how they're, what went well, what didn't go well, how the planning is happening, and sometimes to sort of just, like, drop in like small encouragements, like, evidence of other, I mean I'm far from alone in this, there are other people who are interested in caring and are specifically interested in this thing, or this approach, or this idea that you're rolling around, it can be ideas. (Verity)

Ambiguous fat activism can be provocative and it upsets notions of propriety, purpose and progression in activism. Julia speaks of a period in her life where she took off her clothes in public, an act which often alarmed those around her. She described these moments as early forays into fat activism, later channelled into performance and burlesque, and influenced by the singer Beth Ditto, who has also used public nudity as a fat activist strategy.

I was quite into tearing my clothes off at, like, gigs and parties and things like that, part of, like, when I was being in my element, or whatever the phrase would be, feeling in your element, something like that, would be I'd be like "Woo hoo!" and prance around in my–, and I'd get some–, it would be very unusual for me to get a positive response, I think most people, I mean even my friends, their response would be kind of like feeling protective towards me [mouths something, laughter] [...] and actually like coming up and giving me clothing and "Why don't you put this on?" I think, like, feeling protective of me as like a fat person in their underwear who appeared to not–, I guess they thought like "Oh, she doesn't know what she's doing" or something, I don't know, I guess that was how they read it more, "Oh dear she got so drunk she thinks that's a good idea" or something like that. (Julia)

Julia appeared to be embracing an activist strategy of putting a fat body in a situation where it might appear out of place. She was alone and her intention was uncertain, yet it was still a provocative action about fat, sexuality, and public bodies, so it remains fat activism. The mischievous act of taking off her clothes demanded attention for hers and perhaps other fat women's bodies in contexts where they may have been denigrated or made invisible. But this invites thoughts about the kinds of visibility fat women might want. The intervention was fun for Julia and also generated anxiety and confusion in others. Other fat activists in the sample mentioned lying and vandalism as strategies, which raise ethical issues and produce similarly ambiguous interventions. Ambiguous fat activism emerges when it is produced by people who are "failed" or "less-than ideal" fat activists. Liz described this group:

But most people still don't want to be fat, even if they don't want to engage in a diet culture or engage in a culture that is telling them that they're bad, so they don't want to be viewed as, you know, bad, but they don't really know how to view this kind of idea, issue, outside of their own particular body, and I think fat

activism doesn't do a great job of framing the issue and addressing
that conflict. Because what people often feel like they have to do
in fat activism is be perfect. Fat activists always love their body,
no matter what size it is, always want to be fat, never ever want
to change, and you know, that's the rules. So if that's like, if that's
not how you feel then you can't be a fat activist. And that's the
problem. (Liz)

Where other forms of fat activism exalt good citizenship, the ability to
get along, self-love and mutual respect, ambiguous fat activism is not
immediately or obviously invested in playing fairly or nicely, or wanting
to play at all.

The delights of anti-social behaviour and fat activism are touched
upon by Kathleen LeBesco.[55] Refusing to observe the rules of obesity
discourse unlocks creative, non-conformist and unruly spaces for
revolting fat bodies. W. Charisse Goodman warns that revenge should
not be a motivation for fat activism but Heather MacAllister's menacing
barbeque in front of a weight loss centre smacks of the glee in getting
your own back whether or not this is the good, right or nice thing to
do.[56] Two photo blogs instigated by Substantia Jones also take pleasure
in retaliation and belligerence: *SmileSizeist* invites fat people to take
photographs of their fatphobic harassers, and *FatPeopleFlippingYouOff* is

---

55 LeBesco, *Revolting Bodies.*
56 W. Charisse Goodman, *The Invisible Woman: Confronting Weight Prejudice in America* (Carlsbad CA: Gurze Books, 1995); Charlotte Cooper, "Fat Activism in Ten Astonishing, Beguiling, Inspiring and Beautiful Episodes" in *Fat Studies in the Uk*, edited by Corinna Tomrley and Ann Kaloski Naylor, 19-31 (York: Raw Nerve Books, 2009). Look up The Galactic Acetic Acid Liberation Front, who released a noxious substance in a gallery to protest a fatphobic Mardi Gras poster! The Galactic Acetic Acid Liberation Front, "Fat Fear," *Off Our Backs* 9, no. 4 (1979): 18. See also Kimberly Brittingham who, in a similarly prankish and irreverent vein, made a dummy self-help book cover stating *Fat Is Contagious: How Sitting Next to a Fat Person Can make YOU Fat.* She sat close to people on the New York subway and documented their reactions online. Kimberly Brittingham, "Fat Is Contagious." http://www.freshyarn.com/42/essays/brittingham_fat1.htm.

a repository of images of fat people making obscene and defiant gestures.[57] Elsewhere the anti-social arises in fat activism that is predicated on bullying, particularly in online spaces. Such bullying represents a closed system of community life in which dissent is extremely risky. I will discuss shunning later on, but for now I want to acknowledge that anti-social and ambiguous fat activism – indeed all forms of activism – prompts questions about ethics and harm.

Fun is an important quality of ambiguous fat activism and also appears in disruptive or anti-social interventions. Fun itself might be thought of as activism of an ambiguous kind, perhaps other affective states are too. Whilst Åsa Wettergren claims that anger or outrage are understood as prompts for social action, she also proposes that that fun tends to be neglected even though it generates a feeling of liberation, social cohesion, and basically makes people happy.[58] Joy, pleasure and laughter were referenced many times by the study sample, contrasting sharply with depictions of fatness in obesity discourse, which use humour to diminish or ridicule fat embodiment, or grim accounts of fatphobia. Ashley recalled the uplifting emotional effect of a series of events at the 2009 London Lesbian and Gay Film Festival, one of which being a film show and talk I co-organised.

> I have to say that weekend was like one of the most amazing weekends of my life. I just remember coming to that and going to The Raincoats screening the night before and then Unskinny Bop at the BFI [British Film Institute] and dancing round the hall, and then coming to The Chubsters which I'd convinced [my friend] to come along to with me, actually, and the two of us, who, I'd sort of been thinking a lot about and posting on *Fatshionista* and we'd talked about it, but it being the first, just the most like liberating experience and how that, you know, I remember we

57 Substantia Jones, "Smilesizeist," http://smilesizeist.tumblr.com/; Substantia Jones, "Fatpeopleflippingyouoff," http://fatpeopleflippingyouoff.tumblr.com/.
58 Åsa Wettergren, "Fun and Laughter: Culture Jamming and the Emotional Regime of Late Capitalism," *Social Movement Studies* 8, no. 1 (2009): 1-10.

both came away from it and, er, we came out into the foyer and we were literally so giddy that we span each other around immediately outside. And then I sort of ran off to get the train and I remember sitting on the train back and not being able to sit still and just thinking constantly. Yeah, it really was amazing and I think I came home and shared as many of the films that I could find again on YouTube and whatnot to everyone I knew and, yeah, it was really amazing. (Ashley)

Here fat people were not only recognised and allowed to exist but encouraged to misbehave, dance and thrive through the joyful and mischievous takeover of an institution.

I was interested in how ambiguous fat activism disrupted things that people I have talked to about activism, and whose writing I have read, take for granted about the work of social change. This echoes the struggles with legitimacy that some of the research sample described in referring to micro activism. For example, in their influential book about third wave feminist activism, Jennifer Baumgardner and Amy Richards argue that activism takes place in the everyday and adds up to more substantial social change.[59] But, according to the authors, these acts must include a certain amount of efficiency, accountability, public-ness and impact in order to be thought of as activism. They go on to state that protest "without any constituency" is not activism, but provide no robust evidence for this claim.[60] The problem with this argument is that it creates too narrow a definition of activism, and a result of this is that phenomena that falls outside its boundary is dismissed too quickly as illegitimate.

In a similar vein, I have noticed that there is an inbuilt defensiveness when conveying fat activism to others, it is a preposterous activism that suffers collective low self-esteem because it is regularly subjected

59 Jennifer Baumgardner and Amy Richards, *Manifesta: Young Women, Feminism and the Future* (New York: Farrar, Straus and Giroux, 2000).
60 Baumgardner and Richards, *Manifesta: Young Women, Feminism and the Future*, 283.

to ridicule and attack. Zoë Meleo-Erwin defines fat activism in slightly apologetic tones:

> Of course, fat activism is not a coherent social movement, per se, and rather can be seen as the diverse collection of activist groups, organizations, events, clubs, researchers, websites, internet forums, legal actions, bloggers, zine makers, amongst others, that at a very minimum agree upon the need to challenge anti-fat bias and stereotypes.[61]

But it is a disservice to claim that fat activism must be intelligible to an unnamed other on unnamed terms, or have a universal agenda of challenging stigma and discrimination, in order to earn recognition as a social movement. Indeed, I have shown that fat activism *is* a coherent social movement, it is one that uses many strategies and operates on infinite fronts. In addition, fat activism does not have to be coherent in order to be valid. In not fitting traditional or well-documented forms of social action, fat activism is creating and reflecting new styles of generating social change.

Models that constrain social action leave no space for that which is vague, haphazard, ridiculous, purely about fun, opportunist, multiple, irrational, produced by lone wolves and loose cannons, anti-social or contradictory, yet these qualities exist in fat activism and in other activisms.[62] Elizabeth Armstrong and Mary Bernstein call this an "awkward social movement" because it does not fit pre-existing theory.[63] Rosemary McKechnie and Barbara Körner suggest that activists change

---

61 Zoë Meleo-Erwin, "Disrupting Normal: Toward the 'Ordinary and Familiar' in Fat Politics," *Feminism & Psychology* 22, no. 3 (2012): 1-15.

62 The Mad Pride movement springs to mind as a space where such activism is commonplace. Ted Curtis et al, *Mad Pride: A Celebration of Mad Culture* (London: Spare Change Books, 2000); Robert Deller, *Splitting in Two: Mad Pride and Punk Rock Oblivion* (London: Unkant Publishers, 2014).

63 Elizabeth A. Armstrong and Mary Bernstein, "Culture, Power, and Institutions: A Multi-Institutional Politics Approach to Social Movements," *Sociological Theory* 26, no. 1 (2008): 74-99.

over time and become less certain about what they are doing and more amenable to complexity and ambiguity.[64] Alan Touraine proposes that social movements themselves shift over time because, as Charles Tilly explains, they are of their time.[65] Therefore, social movements that are slippery and fragmented come from cultures that are also mutating, for example through globalisation, the end of communism, global ideological shifts, and the rise of corporations.[66] Moreover, as citizenship becomes more unfixed and migratory, so does activism.[67] Ambiguous fat activism may be a bit peculiar but it is clearly part of a broader repertoire of activism and should not be discounted because most social movement theory has yet to catch up with it. It is clear that everyone is not on the same page regarding how to do fat activism, and neither do they have to be, nobody is in charge of it. This awkward ambiguity is intriguing precisely because it upsets the idea that activism has a fixed meaning with solid boundaries.[68]

In contrast to Baumgardner and Richards' closed definition, ambiguous and immaterial fat activism hint that activism might be a less restricted phenomenon than is generally theorised. I have shown how notions of legitimacy and illegitimacy in fat activism marginalise some forms of action and elevate others, and that activists sometimes do not recognise what they do as activism, or lack confidence in it, because they do not consider it valid. Yet it is my central argument in this chapter that fat activism covers a range of interventions and that many different activities can be thought of as activism. Its effects might be difficult to quantify

64 Rosemary McKechnie and Barbara Körner, "Unruly Narratives: Discovering the Active Self" in *Narrative, Memory and Identities*, edited by David Robinson et al, 67-75 (Huddersfield: University of Huddersfield, 2009).

65 Touraine, "On the Frontier of Social Movements"; Charles Tilly, *Social Movements, 1768-2004* (Boulder, CO: Paradigm Publishers, 2004).

66 Michel Wieviorka, "After New Social Movements," *Social Movement Studies* 4, no. 1 (2005): 1-19.

67 Engin F. Isin, "Citizenship in Flux: The Figure of the Activist Citizen," *Subjectivity*, no. 29 (2009): 367-88.

68 Tilly, *Social Movements, 1768-2004*; Donatella Della Porta and Mario Diani, *Social Movements: An Introduction*, Second edition (Oxford: Blackwell, 2006).

but at the very least it helps generate Butler's liveable lives.[69] If the act of imagining something can be thought of as activism, as Verity proposed above, activism is potentially limitless, beyond boundaries and control, it reveals and implicitly critiques where power materialises and is available to anyone to use it as they like.

A META SOCIAL MOVEMENT

I think of fat activism as a meta social movement because it exists on its own terms but it also offers clues about how other people in other social movements might approach social justice and transformation.

The diversity of fat activism is immense, even amongst a small sample of people connected within a social network. Fat activism is a radical social movement because it is not easily compartmentalised, it bleeds through many boundaries, it has many interests. Fat activism cannot conform, it is uncontainable. There isn't one distinct set of aims. It offers infinite ways of being an activist and shows that activism can be anything: a thought, a decision, a performance, the whole works. The many fat activist methods suggests that there is also a variety of reasons why people pursue fat activism. Sometimes the reasons that people do fat activism are clear, but often they are not, especially in fat activism that goes wrong or is poorly conceived. It is radical because it disrupts the idea that activism can only take place in certain spaces by certain people for particular ends. It is accessible and has the capacity to transform people who would never otherwise be invested in social change into social justice agents.

Social movement theory remains fairly limited in relation to fat activism, but it is still useful to think of fat activism as a social movement because it has the potential to expose the inadequacies of obesity discourse, it shows that fat is more complex than medicalisation or social

69 Butler, *Undoing Gender*; Judith Butler, *Precarious Life: The Powers of Mourning and Violence* (London: Verso, 2004).

pathology and invites other ways of approaching the subject. I have argued that political process fat activism is dominant because this is the type of action most understandable as activism in the 21st century West, not because it is more legitimate than the activism of, for example, arranging a home in which you are comfortably fat.

Meanwhile, proxies for fat activism continue to render it static, as though it never changes or reflects the concerns of particular spaces. It is these mutations over time and place that I will explore in the following chapters.

LOCATING

This chapter begins with me. It's about how I came to fat activism through a particular genealogy of fat feminism which still informs how I think about fat activism. I offer these autoethnographic moments to show that I did not arrive into fat activism fully formed and self-made. I am a social being influenced by things around me and with the potential to influence others, like everybody else. I'm part of a continuum, a series of precedents, a genealogy, I'm a person in time and of place. There is a context for what I think and do and this chapter is all about locating and contextualising what I think of as fat activism. I am writing about myself here, what I am presenting is not *the* history of fat activism, there can never be one history. I want to talk about my own genealogy and encourage others to talk about theirs because I want to show that fat activism is not just a thing that pops up from nowhere, it is embedded in historical, geographical, political and philosophical spaces. It is important to acknowledge this so that fat activists can locate and understand themselves.

In this chapter I will discuss how the fat feminist context that helped form my fat activism came to be overlooked. I will describe where I think it came from and how it looked in the early part of the movement. Many of these stories have not been shared for some time. In sharing them now I hope that they can become a part of an intergenerational transmission of fat activism, an increased focus on historicising the movement, a shift towards greater historiographical sensitivity.[1] But first, here are some things you should know about me.

MY AWAKENING

I was a chubby kid, the daughter of a chubby man and a thin woman who plumped up as she got older. Not everyone in my family is fat, but many of us have a propensity towards fatness which is generally controlled through dieting and compulsive exercise, and sometimes addiction, poverty and abuse. The people in my family do not like or appreciate fatness, it is a source of disgust, failure, shame.

My own fatness started to make an appearance at a time when my working class parents' attempts at trying to pass for middle class colonials were at their height. I wonder if my body seemed like a throwback to them, a betrayal and too revealing in the social circles they wanted to enter.

Around seven or eight years old, my body began to come under scrutiny. One of my siblings became obsessed with my fatness and his relative strength, slenderness and apparent superiority; my body was central to his bullying of me and nobody intervened. My mother began restricting my food. From then until a short while before her death in 1988 when I was 18 we would diet together sporadically. She was a nurse and this would take the form of following eating plans she had brought home from work, usually when Dad was away for extended periods of time. It was a defence against loneliness. We would follow the diets for a week or so and then get bored. I would regain the small amounts of weight I lost. I remember her anxieties that I would never find a boyfriend if I was fat, and bickering in clothes shops where nothing fitted me. I was the only fat person I knew. After she died my dieting intensified for a period. Another sibling pitied me for being fat at this time, a reflection of how I felt about myself. Dad once told me that I looked nice. When he remarried his wife expressed contempt for my body, as have other

---

1 Historiography here means the methods used to create histories.

members of my extended family since then. This scrutiny and anxiety converged on my queer girlhood.

Perhaps because of the surveillance concerning my body, I understood from a young age that fat was something to think and talk about. Confusingly at the time being fat did not prevent me from having friends, being sexual or being physically active. But fat was a factor when I was bullied. It was the source of complaints and comparisons. As a teenager I was joined in these concerns by other girls and so we began to talk about fat together. Around this time I was encountering punk and feminism for the first time. I shaved and dyed my hair. I became involved in anti-fascist student activism. My eldest brother was part of an autonomous community of travellers who lived precariously and unconventionally, I was a frequent visitor to his world. I began to meet queers and trans people. I went out at night. My family was breaking down. I was learning that life might offer other possibilities and that the world of straight people, the normals, was overrated. These ideas remain central to me and I realise now that they produced a rich foundation for thinking about fat in ways that were not otherwise prescribed.

In 1989 I was living in Aberystwyth, bereaved and depressed, in a dismal long distance relationship with a man who pestered me to lose weight. Like many, I picked up a copy of *Fat Is A Feminist Issue* because of its title, hoping to discover why my body was seemingly such a problem. But I did not find answers there, instead I felt shamed by the assumption that my fatness was pathological and it took me a long time to release myself from its grip. For a while I was stuck.

Although there were many threads to my politicisation, it was an episode of the long departed BBC talk show *Wogan* that formed my epiphany.[2] It seems very strange to me now that this unlikely location could have been so influential. I have not seen this programme since it was broadcast but I remember the host interviewing perhaps two women from the London Fat Women's Group about their forthcoming conference. I also watched the group's BBC *Open Space* documentary, a

2 BBC, *Wogan*, UK, 1989. Television.

community programme in which they had editorial control, broadcast at prime time.³ I was now aware that British feminists were writing and organising around fat differently to those who came at it from an interest in eating disorders although at the time I couldn't tell the difference, I just knew that it spoke to me. These were actual fat women, they had an analysis of fat oppression, they were a community. I felt as though the women were speaking about my experience and I watched them hungrily.

I became a vegetarian and learned to cook for and nourish myself, but I still experienced sporadic attempts to lose weight by restricting my eating. Gradually this stopped though I continued to buy diet versions of food and thought of exercise as a tool to help me control how I looked. By the early 1990s these habits petered out, partly because I began a relationship with someone who loved me and I saw no reason to carry on with what was plainly self-destructive behaviour, and mostly because I had started to develop my thoughts around fat and apply them to my life; I was getting politicised.

UNDERSTANDING CONTEXTS

I asked people I interviewed for this project how they came to be fat activists and although the content of the stories varied, there were similarities in the form and process. We all experienced moments where we had been made into a problem by others; we had realisations about this that occurred through series of events; these events led to shifts over time, like a dot-to-dot picture that slowly reveals itself. I noticed that in the telling, people were keen to share their autobiographies but that theorising did not take place, a position also argued by Hannele Harjunen.⁴ Participants who did suggest theoretical rationales for what they do tended to offer very broad explanations at a high level of abstraction than more specific comments.

3 BBC, *Fat Women Here to Stay*, *Open Space*, UK, 1989. Television.
4 Harjunen, *Women and Fat: Approaches to the Social Study of Fatness.*

And I've always been interested in the body, and how we construct the body and what the body means as fat people and how we perform our embodiment as fat people. (Kris)

A lot of it is about visibility and putting fat bodies on stage. (Daniah)

Leora was unusual in that she related her earliest encounters with fat activism to feminism and queer sex:

> You know I think that I first really felt and appreciated [fat activism] and was aware of it was with my first real fat lover, even though I had had crushes on other fat people. And so, you know the fact that she was so politicised and also it was so hot, was really mind-blowing and it just, you know, was a very different, it was different to feel that that was an integrated part of what made me sexy, and also it was just really a good place in time to be, you know, around all of these other fat freaks, and I feel that that really revolutionised me, I have no idea what would have happened if that hadn't happened, really. I can't even imagine!

> Charlotte: So that was, I mean had you heard about fat activism before you met your first real fat lover at all?

> I had not. You know it was certainly not about fat activism from lesbians, and I had never heard of the Fat Underground, and I had very little idea of any kind of history around it, and I think that the closest I had ever come was *Fat Is A Feminist issue*, and that was a little bit of a not revolutionary read for me, not all that politicised for being such a political statement. So, you know, I will say that there were some peripheral things that I feel like I had learned for body acceptance in other parts of feminism, and that feminism and feminist work really did make a lot more room for different kinds of abilities and body types and shapes to

be acceptable, and I was really raised by feminists, and I feel like, you know, I was raised by somebody who didn't feel like hairy armpits were freaky and but that I should be ashamed of myself for pointing and staring, you know! And I was, you know. But I don't feel that specifically, it was this violent thing, body and size acceptance. (Leora)

I wondered if it was difficult for people to identify how they were brought into being as fat activists in terms of their foundational ideas, beliefs, values, politics and so on.[5] For example, there were moments in the research interviews for this project where people were talking about things that I had instigated that had influenced them, but they did not refer to this. It was as though they had magically come across these things by themselves. This was very subtle, only I would know the origins of what they were talking about and I didn't comment because I didn't want to appear big-headed. I doubted myself too, perhaps I was failing to recognise people's agency, maybe I wasn't as original as I'd hoped to be. I know that I do not always manage to give credit for things that have influenced me. Nevertheless, I noted this hesitation around naming and locating contexts.[6]

I became curious about the things that bound the diverse sample for this research together. It felt as though we were talking about similar things without specifying those similarities. Discourse was well-integrated into people's lives but I wanted to separate it out again, to be explicit about it so that we could take a good look at ourselves. I wanted to understand fat activist ancestries and think about how they relate to current and future concerns within the movement. I thought that doing this would reveal new sites for action and areas for critical enquiry and deepen understanding of the movement. There are consequences

5 "Discursively produced" in academic jargon.
6 It led me to reflect on what contextualising oneself might mean for fat activists. Where people have managed to transform abjection into something more positive through their fat activism or through an activist identity and persona, it might be difficult, humbling or painful to acknowledge that you are one of many rather than entirely unique or exceptional.

when fat activist contexts are ignored or denied because they are seen as ephemeral or documented obscurely.

FAT FEMINISM

Just as there is no single fat activism, there is no single origin story. There are countless genealogies of fat activism, not all of which are feminist.[7] But I want to talk about the first discourse I encountered that helped me make sense of my fatness, my ancestries, namely a fat feminism that started in the US.[8] In 1989 this was where fat was understood explicitly and meaningfully to me as part of a matrix of power, gender and sexuality. I remain with it today for these reasons, because it is sophisticated and because it articulates, and continues to illuminate, the massive contributions by women, especially queers, lesbians and bisexual women, to fat activism and to activism in general.[9] The problems within feminism, its struggles around race, imperialism, trans people, or class for example, also reflect problems within fat activism and perhaps offer some ways of addressing these issues. Fat feminism plays an important role in how I experience fat activist community and how I found the people who I interviewed for this project. I make this claim on the basis that some of the study participants were part of fat feminist interventions in the 1970s and

7 For example, Zora Simic locates fat feminist origins in the mid-19th century dress reform movement rather than civil rights, as I have done here. Zora Simic, "Fat as a Feminist Issue: A History" in *Fat Sex: New Directions in Theory and Activism*, edited by Helen; Hester and Caroline Walters, 15-35 (Farnham: Ashgate, 2015). Fat activism based in sex and fetish cultures is not always feminist. For example *Dimensions* magazine, published in print between 1984 and 2004, now an online forum. Anonymous, "Dimensions." http://www.dimensionsmagazine.com/.

8 Throughout this book, when I mention fat feminism it is this specific genealogy to which I am referring though I tend to use the generic 'fat feminism' in the text.

9 Indeed, Esther Rothblum proposes that lesbians lead the way in showing the general population how to develop fat self-acceptance. Esther D. Rothblum, "Commentary: Lesbians Should Take the Lead in Removing the Stigma That Has Long Been Associated with Body Weight," *Psychology of Sexual Orientation and Gender Diversity* (2014): 1-6.

1980s. Others participated in projects that bridged fat feminist and fat queer feminist activist communities a decade later. Some research participants came to fat activism as a result of knowing me and reading my work, and some younger contributors found fat activism through a strand of Fat Studies that has uninterrupted genealogical connections to fat feminism. A small number were feminists allied to queer theory and practice who incorporated their fat activism into that framework, and have since developed a synthesis of fat queer feminism.

What follows is a discussion of how this particular strand of fat feminism has come to be overlooked, and then a mapping-out of some of its origins.

WHY FAT FEMINISM IS OBSCURE

The fat feminism I am talking about here pre-dates the feminist proxies for fat activism that I mentioned previously. It is a feminist activist analysis of fat based on lived and shared experience rather than secondary accounts, theory or research. With these credentials one would think it would be well-known and highly valued but it is not, and here are some suggestions for why this is so.

Fragile historicising

At the moment it is rare for fat activists to share historical information with each other, and intergenerational spaces are thin on the ground. Knowledge is feebly documented and preserved, it is not passed on and it is hard to find unless you know where to look, there is no outreach. There are few repositories and no network to guide people to those collections. Where *Fat Is A Feminist Issue* has gone through many editions, fat feminist texts tend to be buried deep within archives. These institutions are not always accessible, collections may be thousands of miles away from where you live, and subject to arcane admission criteria. Archives are also vulnerable to funding lapses or collapse, as happened to Largesse, an online fat feminist archive that contained invaluable scanned copies of original Fat Underground documents.

Political rifts

Part of the difficulty in reasserting fat feminism is that it is stems from the "wrong kind of feminism." The feminism that supported early fat activism is not fashionable and is problematic in its approach to contemporary feminist concerns around gender and sex. It is likely that this inhibits many activists, especially those working within anti-oppression frames, from engaging with a feminism that has oppressive aspects. It also inhibits the intergenerational transmission of fat feminism between feminists who come from different traditions. Although radical lesbian feminism incubated fat activism historically, these ties now seem broken. Even within contemporary sex worker- and trans- exclusionary radical lesbian feminist politics, fat activism is marginalised as a possible site of resistance. There is an absence of historical continuation from fat feminism and earlier radical feminism. For example, Sheila Jeffreys' work on beauty and gender makes no reference to fat activism and reproduces a pretty standard academic take on bodies and patriarchy.[10]

Occupation

I have written that Orbach is a figure of frustration for fat activists but she symbolises a broader exasperation about a lack of feminist engagement with fat activism.[11] Fat feminism has suffered an occupation. I am using the metaphor of occupation because it has been dominated and obscured by some feminists and this has had a negative impact on the actions of fat feminist activists. For example it has been used to justify and reproduce fat hatred, as experienced by Ashley:

10 Sheila Jeffreys, *Beauty and Misogyny: Harmful Cultural Practices in the West* (London: Routledge, 2005).
11 Aldebaran, "Letter: Oob Perpetuating Stereotypes," *Off Our Backs* 9, no. 11 (1979): 31.

I remember going to see a potential PhD supervisor when I was finishing my MA, and her kind of talking about fat activism and saying: "Yes, it's all fine and great for people like you because, you know, like, you look nice and are perfectly acceptable, but you know there's a point, isn't there, and you know, obviously I support you but I wouldn't necessarily support someone who's a size 30 or something," I believe was close to what she said. [...] And, I think it's that sort of hypocrisy that comes with certain types of body activism and body, and particularly, like, feminist body work, that annoys me more than anything else. (Ashley)

What Ashley describes as hypocrisy also emerges elsewhere in lesbian feminist writing about fat.[12] In addition, feminist preoccupation with eating disorders that lacks an analysis of fat hatred has been used to intrude on fat activist spaces and undermine them. For example, Kate Moran describes its destructive effects on the radical lesbian feminist cultures that incubated fat feminism as a discourse central to the 12-step recovery programme Overeaters Anonymous (OA):

There is nowhere in the lesbian community where fat lesbians are safe from the proselytising zealots of OA. They pester fat lesbians individually at lesbian events or publicly at parties, where it is especially humiliating as a fat lesbian to try and prove you do not compulsively overeat. They have broken up fat support groups in Oasis at the Michigan Womyn's Music Festival in 1984; the year before, at the same festival, they interrupted Fat Liberation workshops. Linda Tillery and Maxine Feldman have both spoken from the main stage at Michigan about how they look great now

12 See for example Tamsin Wilton's filtering of obesity discourse through lesbian feminist health models. She insists that discrimination against anyone on the basis of looks is unacceptable, but claims again that fat is a problematic result of faulty eating and bad psychology and that fat activism is a misguided attempt to engender power by becoming physically bigger than men! Tamsin Wilton, *Good for You: A Handbook of Lesbian Health and Wellbeing* (London: Cassell, 1997).

due to their amazing recoveries in OA. Lesbians have fought with the Michigan Festival for years to get good-looking festival t-shirts and sportswear in large sizes; some years there are one or two t-shirt styles, some years there is nothing. But you can count on six OA meetings a day and all the sprouts you can eat.[13]

Of continuing aggravation to fat activists is that this occupying discourse supports the idea that fat should be primarily theorised and developed by normatively-sized people without consulting fat people.

> Why are they thinking about this all the time through the experience of the thin woman? Why is fat never mentioned or people who are more or less permanently fat? Where are they in this picture? And they weren't anywhere. (Impi)

It is infuriating to fat activists, including some of the research sample, that normatively-embodied feminists have attempted to claim authorship and ownership of fat experience. Other fat feminists, vexed by its lack of visibility and occupied status, have attempted to draw attention to this older fat feminism,[14] with limited results. Excavating this older fat feminism is an act of reclaiming it from occupation, making it available for discussion and re-stating the centrality of fat people's experience.

---

13 Kate Moran, "One Step Forward, Two Steps Back: Fat Liberation and Overeaters Anonymous" in *Dossier: Oppression De La Grosseur*, edited by Danielle Charest et al, 103-12 (Montréal: Amazones d'Hier, Lesbiennes d'Aujourdhui, 1992). Marjory Nelson offers a similar fat feminist critique of OA that pre-dates Moran by nine years. Marjory Nelson, "Letter: Thinly Veiled Insult," *Off Our Backs* 13, no. 5 (1983): 30.

14 Elly Janesdaughter, "Letter: Fatophobic Feminists," *Off Our Backs* 9, no. 7 (1979): 28; Jenkins and Smith, "Fat Liberation."

SOME STARTING POINTS

A less than meagre scholarly literature on early fat feminism means that the origin story I am presenting is a scavenging expedition centred on encounters with the archive. It is an assemblage of scattered resources, texts of forgetfulness and omission, contingent and forever incomplete. As I produce this story I am mindful of the literature on the slippery nature of social memory and narrative.[15] But I have not been able to count on others to tell this story. Instead, this assemblage consists of activist encounters with archives of fat activism: it is my direct experience of fat activist communities over many years that has enabled me to navigate obscure physical and virtual repositories, embark on personal communications and oral histories, solicit accounts by people in the sample who contributed to the movement's origins, and participate in the collective conversational acts of remembering and noting.[16] The act of assembling an archive of my fat feminist origins is also rendered here as activism, a resource from which to develop critical awareness. I used to think of these origins as waves contiguous with the theorising of feminism in wave forms, but I have changed my mind since then because the threads of fat feminism cannot be neatly contained within that structure, they are not always linear but continuous and interweaving.[17]

15 Francesca Polletta, "Contending Stories: Narrative in Social Movements," *Qualitative Sociology* 21, no. 4 (1998): 419-46; Barbara A. Misztal, *Theories of Social Remembering* (Maidenhead: Open University Press, 2003); Maria G. Cattell and Jacob G. Climo, "Introduction: Meaning in Social Memory and History: Anthropological Perspectives" in *Social Memory and History: Anthropological Perspectives*, edited by Jacob G. Climo and Maria G. Cattell, 1-38 (Walnut Creek, CA: AltaMira Press, 2002); Shari Stone-Mediatore, *Reading Across Borders: Storytelling and Knowledges of Resistance* (New York: Palgrave Macmillan, 2003).

16 Cooper, "A Queer and Trans Fat Activist Timeline-Zine Download"; Charlotte Cooper, "A Queer and Trans Fat Activist Timeline: Queering Fat Activist Nationality and Cultural Imperialism," *Fat Studies: An Interdisciplinary Journal of Body Weight and Society* 1, no. 1 (2012): 61-74.

17 Charlotte Cooper, "Fat Studies: Mapping the Field," *Sociology Compass* 4, no. 12 (2010): 1020-34; Deborah M. Withers, "Strategic Affinities: Historiography and

THE FAT-IN

The first documented example of a fat activist moment that I could find, and which has ties to the genealogy that I am about to unfurl, has the hallmarks of an elaborate prank as well as elements of sincerity. It took place on 3 June 1967 at Sheep Meadow, in New York's Central Park.

The Fat-In was the idea of Steve Post, a radio host at the WBAI station.[18] The Fat-In followed on the heels of other contemporary countercultural gatherings, such as the Fly-In, the Sweep-In, both produced by his colleague Bob Fass, and the Be-In.[19]

Post helped pioneer a style of broadcasting known as free radio, and the Fat-In was an event that helped bring him to prominence as a proponent of confessional, conversational, irreverent and spontaneous interactions with listeners. Post had grown into a normatively-sized adult but was previously a fat child who suffered from poor self-esteem. The Fat-In was initiated after Post read what he thought was a generic article in *The New York Times Magazine* about the social struggles of fat children, bordered with advertisements for chocolate cake and weight loss. He felt that this juxtaposition illustrated the impossible social positioning of fat children and of fat people, as well as the contradictory ways in which consumption and weight loss were sold. He fantasised about a group coming together to rid themselves of fat hatred and come out as fat. He proposed that such an event could be called a Fat-In and that they should use the slogan "Fat Power," allying the event with other liberation movements of the time. He started to talk about it on air and it soon became a hot topic. Post's listeners shared their own stories of fat oppression, developed a philosophy of Fat Power and, as a result of

Epistemology in Contemporary Feminist Knowledge Politics," *European Journal of Women's Studies* 22, no. 2 (2015): 129-42.

18 WBAI is not an acronym, simply the call sign for the station, although it does refer to the station's previous owners, Broadcast Associates Incorporated.

19 Steve Post, *Playing in the Fm Band: A Personal Account of Free Radio* (New York: The Viking Press, 1974); Jeff Land, "Pacifica's Wbai: Free Radio and the Claims of Community," *Jump Cut* 41 (1997): 93-101.

this, he decided to make the event a reality.

Post reported that about 500 people of all sizes came to the Fat-In. Some used clothing to express their disdain for weight loss, flaunting themselves in horizontal stripes (long regarded in popular culture as a fashion no-no for fat people), too tight garments and tape measure belts. Banners and badges included the slogans: "Fat Power," "Buddha Was Fat," "Take a Fat Girl to Dinner," and "Help Cure Emaciation".[20] People ate forbidden junk food together[21] and the climax of the event was a burning of a life-sized photograph of the model Twiggy, who represented to Post the symbolic elevation of thinness above all else. The Fat-In garnered extensive publicity through syndicated news reports in New York, California, Wisconsin and Montana[22] and brought new audiences to WBAI, although some of Post's management at the station's parent company Pacifica were unimpressed.

The Fat-In was a protest against fat hatred and looks a lot like some of the activism that I have produced, particularly the Fattylympics, as well as offering the qualities of ambiguous activism that I discussed in the previous chapter. I would argue that it owes a debt to the spectacle and unruliness of Situationism as well as Mikhail Bhakhtin's theories of the carnivalesque.[23] On other occasions where I have written about the Fat-In I have assumed it was more of a joke than a genuine attempt to create a public discussion of fat with subversive humour. This is due to the paucity of documentary evidence surrounding it and my reliance

20 Anonymous, "Food for Thought," *Sports Illustrated*, 19 June 1967, 12.

21 A strategy that has continued on occasion. See, for example, how young fat activists of colour have used junk food and communal eating in this way in Marty Fink's article referencing the *It Gets Fatter* project in Toronto. Fink, "It Gets Fatter: Graphic Fatness and Resilient Eating in Mariko and Jillian Tamaki's Skim." Other fat activists write about their entitlement to enjoy food as much as anybody else. Katie D., "Rolls with Butter: A Fat Activist Zine," n.d.

22 Anonymous, "Curves Have Their Day in Park; 500 at a 'Fat-in' Call for Obesity" *New York Times*, 5 June 1967.

23 Guy Debord, *The Society of the Spectacle* (St Petersburg FL: Black & Red, 1984); Mikhail Bakhtin, *Rabelais and His World* (Bloomington, IN: Indiana University Press, 1984).

on mocking newspaper reports. But Post's 1974 account of working in free radio, which surfaced online following his death in 2014, has made me reassess this position. The Fat-In was sincere[24] but there remains some dissent as to whether or not it was fat activism. William Fabrey of NAAFA spoke to Post about the event in 1982 and he later reflected:

> At the time, it was commonplace to seize on any outrageous topic and hold a sit-in, as you point out. Reporters would be sure to show up. It was an attempt to put radio station WBAI before the public. Participants sometimes barely knew what they were protesting – it was the 'camp' thing to do. I heard that Post himself was a compulsive dieter for years after that. Nonetheless, the event was noteworthy on its own merits. But it had no steam behind it.[25]

Fabrey, whose own activism was initially built on his attraction to fat women, illustrates here the preoccupation with what constitutes *real* activism. But I think he misses the point. The Fat-In *was* the steam, it was a highly influential event and clearly contextualised in similar activisms of that time and place. The photo-activist Substantia Jones, who has also worked at WBAI as Kimberley Massengill, commented that Post's reasons for producing the Fat-In may have been self-serving and satirical, but his work had a lasting effect of which few present-day fat activists are aware.[26] Nevertheless, the event is not beyond critique. Jones refers to the burning of Twiggy's photograph as an act of

24 As far as I know, Post did not continue have a public life around fat politics and few obituaries mentioned the *Fat-In*. But it is likely the event remained personally important. On 20 March 2015, what would have been Post's birthday, a memorial was held for him at Symphony Space on the Upper West Side of New York City. On the podium, according to picture evidence from a friend of a friend who was there, was his Fat Power placard from the *Fat-In*.

25 W.J. Fabrey, email, 4 January 2009.

26 David Hinckley, "New York Radio Contrarian and Wnyc Morning Host Steve Post Dies at Age 70." http://www.nydailynews.com/entertainment/new-york-radio-show-host-steve-post-dies-age-70-article-1.1890789.

body-shaming that would not be acceptable today, and to this I would add that there are gender implications to that action, one might say misogyny. Anti-feminism was one of the motivations for fat feminism during the early days of fat activism, which I shall now discuss.

NAAFA

Fat feminism became necessary because of the marginalisation of women, including lesbians, feminist and otherwise, within NAAFA, the organisation that is often used as a proxy for fat activism.

The organisation began with Llewellyn (Lew) Louderback, who was a hack writer and journalist from New York.[27] In November 1967 he published an article in *The Saturday Evening Post*, a popular magazine, advocating respect and rights for fat people.[28]

> My motivation for writing the piece was my outrage at the kind of life my wife [Ann] had been forced to live as a fat woman. (She died four years ago. Of lung cancer, of course, since she was a follower of the 'reach for a smoke instead of a sweet' school of weight control).[29]

An engineer called William Fabrey contacted Louderback as a consequence, he wanted to distribute reprints of the article. Fabrey identified then and now as a fat admirer.[30] Although Louderback was fat, it was for the sake of his and Fabrey's wives, Ann Louderback and

27 Llewellyn Louderback, *Operation Moon Rocket [Pseudonym Nick Carter]* (London: Tandem, 1968); Llewellyn Louderback, *Pretty Boy, Baby Face - I Love You* (Philadelphia: Coronet, 1969).

28 Llewellyn Louderback, "More People Should Be Fat," *Saturday Evening Post*, 4 November 1967, 10-12.

29 Llewellyn Louderback, 11 August 2008.

30 Fat admirers are people, generally normatively-sized straight men, who have a sexual preference for fat partners, usually women.

Joyce Fabrey, that they issued a call to action. Together they convened a group of nine people and approved a formal constitution and bylaws for NAAFA, then the National Association to Aid Fat Americans, on 13 June 1969.[31] Fabrey was designated leader and founder of the organisation.

The following year Louderback published *Fat Power*, the title of which references the Fat-In, with research assistance from Ann and the Fabreys.[32]

> Ann did a lot of the research, incidentally, she was working for an ad agency. Her job was editing, proof-reading and getting everything just right on these ads. Terrible pharmaceutical ads. But she had access through the company to all kinds of magazines that she could get articles from.[33]

Fat Power, a lively and accessible read, argues that fat hatred is ingrained in media, medicine, fashion and weight loss industries. Readers are encouraged to resist and critique this, although tactics are not specified beyond a general call for civil rights. Louderback counters claims about fat health and makes reference to fat historical and cultural figures,suggesting that fatness is a concept that can exist beyond the clinic. The book speaks to many of the concerns of the movement today but is also pre-feminist and heteronormative, and its politics are naïve, particularly around race and class. In personal correspondence with me, Louderback revealed that he struggled to publicise the book because the media wanted to poke fun at him. He declined an invitation to appear on *The Johnny Carson Show*, a popular programme, and as a result, the book did not sell as well as he had hoped. Fabrey commented:

> It was a miracle that [*Fat Power*] was published at all. The

31 Fabrey, W. J. "Thirty-Three Years of Size Acceptance in Perspective - How Has It Affected the Lives of Real People?" http://members.tripod.com/~bigastexas/2001event/keynote2001.html.

32 Lew Louderback, *Fat Power* (New York: Hawthorn Books, 1970).

33 Lew Louderback, Personal Correspondence with Author, 20 August 2008.

original publisher, Meredith Press, who had the manuscript sold it, with a batch of others, to Hawthorn Books, I believe, and Hawthorn treated it like an orphan. Only one editor, at the original publisher believed in it, and in Lew, and he or she left the company. Hawthorn's attitude, according to Lew, was "Well, all right, I suppose we have to publish it, but a limited press run, no budget for publicity, and keep the pages to a minimum." What saddened me most was that [Louderback] didn't save the original manuscript, before all the cuts, and especially the footnotes, and that wasn't the publisher's fault.[34]

Louderback left the organisation shortly afterwards.

Fabrey concedes that the people who joined NAAFA were not politicised and the organisation quickly reformulated itself into a series of local social groups, called chapters, and special interest groups. NAAFA became an important institution for many people who would otherwise have been isolated. The organisation also helped to popularise language and concepts unique to the movement: supersized, fat admirer, fat acceptance. According to Fabrey:

> What I actually helped to achieve was a more responsive fashion industry, and a subculture of people who accept themselves, and those who admire them. My being an FA (a term I helped coin) feels a little more mainstream, sort of, than it ever was, but there are still hateful people who will still put me down because of it, and lots of fatphobia out there, as always. But now there is a whole movement to deal with it. I helped to give it a kick-start, although it took about 30 years longer than expected.[35]

Over its lifetime NAAFA has harboured big ambitions and enjoyed a relatively large membership and reach, but has lacked the organisational

---

34 W. J. Fabrey, Email, 10 August 2008.
35 W. J. Fabrey, Email, 4 January 2009.

power to capitalise on its strengths.[36] The earliest structural problems of political naivety combined with an inexperienced and conservative membership were never really resolved, and it remains problematic, for reasons I will outline below, that fat admirers became directors of an organisation in which the objects of their interest needed full autonomy. Nevertheless, NAAFA remains an important touchstone as a very long-standing group advocating for fat people. It is remarkable that it exists at all.

ANTI-FEMINISM

NAAFA was conceived as an organisation by men who have a sexual interest in fat women who were interested in developing activism that benefitted them as well as the fat people to whom they were attracted. Fabrey, who had limited experience of political organising, outlined his aims:

> I wanted to make the world a safer and more pleasant place for persons of size, and for them to like themselves better, and lastly, and less important, for nobody to tell me what my taste should be.[37]

The primacy of men's sexuality has resulted in an organisational culture in NAAFA where men were and are regarded as a scarce and precious resource, as observed by Anna:

> In the conference I went to, I felt that there was a competition for, fierce competition – that's how they're fierce – fierce competition for, like, skinny guys, and a few people doing what I would characterise as activist work, you know, having Elizabeth Fisher with her seatbelt extender campaign, and some of the stuff that Marilyn Wann tried to do when she became a board member. But for the most part it seems like a social scene, and not that I'm

36 Harding, "Dear Naafa".
37 W. J. Fabrey, Email, 10 August 2008.

opposed to a social scene, but it's a little bit boring, and a little bit focused on winning male approval. And I would be equally troubled if it were focused on winning female approval, it's not the maleness necessarily of that dynamic-

Charlotte: It's about the seeking approval.

Yeah. (Anna)

NAAFA established an uncomfortable relationship with the women's liberation movement. The organisation was founded on behalf of Fabrey and Louderback's wives, but both Ann and Joyce, who are now dead, and other women involved in establishing it, are voiceless and generally nameless in accounts. Fabrey attempted to foster strategic relationships with feminism, writing to *Ms* magazine in 1972 to congratulate them on including fat in the matrix of factors for social exclusion, and by inviting Karen Jones to write about sexism for the NAAFA newsletter in 1974.[38] But the organisation's underlying culture did not change. NAAFA created a Fat Feminist Caucus from 1983, but this took nine years to get going because it was consistently blocked by anti-feminist members, and homophobia at board level prevented a number of lesbian fat feminists from gaining recognition until as late as 1987.[39] The Caucus produced a journal, *New Attitude*, edited by Judy Freespirit, and convened a number of gatherings until at least 2000 but it no longer exists. A NAAFA Feminist Special Interest Group existed for some time but its activities are under-documented and inconclusive as far as I could find.

NAAFA's public face was one of social action, but the organisation also functioned as a meeting place for fat women and men who were sexually attracted to them. Although many women members welcome sexual

38 Johnnie Tillmon, "Welfare as a Women's Issue," *Ms.* 1, no. 1 (1972): 111; Karen W. Jones, "Naafa Newsletter: Fat and Female – One Woman's View," www.eskimo.com/~largesse/Archives/Fatfemale.html
39 Karen Stimson, "Fat Feminist Herstory, 1969-1993: A Personal Memoir," http://www.eskimo.com/~largesse/Archives/herstory.html.

attention, NAAFA's founding values also produced a space in which sexual harassment was tolerated. For example, Erich Goode was able to abuse his position as a researcher with impunity, sexually exploiting a number of his informants.[40] Other women attending NAAFA gatherings have complained of non-consensual encounters, like Liat:

> I got in the pool and there was this straight guy with two NAAFA women, you know, one on each side, and I get in the pool and I had a two-piece at the time, and he was like, he like made some comment to me, and I'm like, "Dude, I'm a lesbian." Like, "BACK OFF!" (Liat)

The marginalising of women within NAAFA, the active prevention of their access to organisational power, a patriarchal culture tolerant of sexual harassment, tokenistic attempts to engage with feminism, homophobia and sexism more generally, and a conservative membership base produced an organisation where women not primarily interested in finding male sexual partners could not flourish as political agents.

THE FAT UNDERGROUND

Although there are fat feminists in NAAFA, others seceded at various times. In the early part of the movement they started alternative organisations, the most prominent of which became The Fat Underground.

Formation

Two Jewish feminists living in Los Angeles in the early 1970s, Judy Freespirit and Aldebaran (also known as Vivian F. Mayer and Sara Golda

---

40 Bell, "Sexualizing Research: Response to Erich Goode"; Erich Goode, "Sexual Involvement and Social Research in a Fat Civil Rights Organization,"; Saguy, "Sex, Inequality, and Ethnography: Response to Erich Goode."

Bracha Fishman), were NAAFA members and part of the Radical Feminist Therapy Collective, one of the most powerful, prestigious and visible groups in the radical fringe in Los Angeles at that time.[41] Radical therapy was critical of the medicalisation and de-politicisation of ordinary human experience and oppression, it was a social model of mental health, it sought systemic change, and was based in a Marxist approach to power.[42] Feminist radical therapy included an analysis of gender within this critical understanding of psychiatry and mental health.[43] In 1972 Freespirit and Aldebaran approached the Free University at Berkeley to train in radical psychiatry. They wanted to apply a similar critique to the medicalisation of fat, especially the medical mistreatment of fat people. Lynn Mabel-Lois (later Lynn McAfee), joined them. Aldebaran explains:

> About two years ago [1972] we began to talk between ourselves and to friends to develop an analysis of the oppression of fat women that fitted into the framework of radical therapy: the idea that people are okay, not sick, and that people's crazy and sad feelings come out of living oppressed lives.[44]

In 1973 the women founded a chapter of NAAFA in Los Angeles, but this alliance was fraught. Freespirit commented:

"It was like the Black Panthers working with the NAACP",[45] she

41 Yolanda Retter, "Lesbian Activism in Los Angeles, 1970-1979" in *Queer Frontiers: Millennial Geographies, Genders, and Generations*, edited by Joseph Allen Boone, 196-221 (Madison, WI The University of Wisconsin Press, 2000).
42 Joseph Agel, *The Radical Therapist* (New York: Ballantine Books, 1971).
43 Carolyn Zerbe Enns, *Feminist Theories and Feminist Psychotherapies: Origins, Themes, and Diversity* (Binghampton, NY: Harrington Park Press, 1997).
44 Aldebaran, "1974 Letter from Aldebaran to Karen Jones" in *The Fat Underground: The Original Radical Fat Feminists - a Commemorative Sourcebook from the Archives of Largesse, the Network for Size Esteem*, edited by Karen Stimson, 56-61 (New Haven, CT: Largesse, 1995).
45 National Association for the Advancement of Colored People, an organisation positioned as politically conservative by more radical activists.

says of the old factions within NAAFA. "Their idea of activism was to go to the Cerebral Palsy Foundation and do volunteer work so that people would say that fat people are nice. Ours was to demonstrate – break into a university lecture hall at UCLA during a class on behaviour modification (for weight loss) and take over the classroom."[46]

Martha, who became involved with fat feminism later on, corroborates Freespirit's analogy:

I always used to say that [NAAFA] were the NAACP of fat liberation, which isn't a bad analogy in its own way, and there we were, you know, basically saying, "Tear down the wall motherfucker!" and it's like a very challenging moment. (Martha)

This political rift, not to mention NAAFA's on-going problems with sexism and homophobia, could no longer be reconciled. Fishman commented:

Our confrontational stance eventually drew the attention of NAAFA's main office. Although some of the leadership privately applauded us, officially we were told to tone down our delivery, and also to be more circumspect about our feminist ideology, which most NAAFA members were not yet ready for.[47]

Eventually the women formally withdrew their membership and focused on further synthesising fat politics with feminism.

In November 1973 The Radical Feminist Therapy Collective began a Fat Women's Problem Solving Group at the Westside Women's Centre, which was facilitated by Aldebaran and "Simone, a fat woman who is not in the F.U. (whatever that means at this point)".[48] This was a popular

46 J.E. Relly, "The Big Issue," http://www.tucsonweekly.com/tw/10-01-98/feat.htm.
47 Fishman, "Life in the Fat Underground".
48 Aldebaran, "1974 Letter from Aldebaran to Karen Jones."

"weekly drop-in rap group for women".[49] They produced the document *A Fat Women's Problem-Solving Group: Radical Change* which explains how the group was able to politicise their personal experiences of being fat through discussion and analysis.[50] The Fat Women's Problem Solving Group morphed into The Fat Underground. By 1975 they had a mission statement:

> The Fat Underground confronts the double oppression of fat women in society through our nutritional, psychological and politically radical analyses of our condition which dispute all present myths about fat. Through media appearances, consciousness-raising and informative written materials we provide a support group for fat women who are not dieting and we provide outreach to those who wish to politically align themselves with their fat sisters.[51]

The Fat Underground was technically open to all, but it became known as a women's group for feminists. Other women who were not feminists left the group, as did a man named Ray Simpson, who formed FACT in Pasadena: "Fat Action Coming Together. It's more establishment than FU [Fat Underground], and more activist than NAAFA, or rather, will be".[52] In researching this book I could not verify the outcome of FACT.

Theorising fat oppression

The Fat Underground were the first to theorise fat oppression, a major contribution to the movement. This they did through a combination

49 Vivian F. Mayer, "Foreword" in *Shadow on a Tightrope: Writings by Women on Fat Oppression*, edited by Lisa Schoenfielder and Barb Wieser, ix-xvii (Iowa City: Aunt Lute, 1983).
50 Aldebaran et al, *A Fat Women's Problem-Solving Group: Radical Change* (Los Angeles: The Fat Underground/Largesse Fat Liberation Archives, n.d.)
51 The Fat Underground, "Introduction to Fat Underground and Radical Feminist Therapy Collective, from Women's Center Brochure," http://web.archive.org/web/20070808155443/http://www.largesse.net/Archives/FU/women'scenter.html.
52 Aldebaran, "1974 Letter from Aldebaran to Karen Jones."

of ideas, action and innovative strategies. They used feminism as a theoretical basis for their activism in four central areas.

Firstly, Louderback's *Fat Power* inspired the formation of The Fat Underground by spelling out a terrain of fatphobia, but Mayer notes: "Louderback's analysis of why the oppression exists was sketchy".[53] Freespirit and Aldebaran's *Fat Liberation Manifesto* locates fat embodiment within a wider social context, identifies the humanity of fat people, and encourages them to claim rights, autonomy and collective power within a framework of commercial and medical exploitation, named as "special enemies", whose interests are supported by unethical and erroneous obesity science.[54] Twenty-five years after publishing the manifesto, Fishman remarks that their alliances with other struggles, including those against racism, capitalism and imperialism is what made their analysis extraordinary. Fat was no longer a site for personal failing and redemption but was reconfigured and aligned within a political landscape.[55] Although The Fat Underground were of the left, the left "neither wanted or accepted us" and despite their willingness to develop wide-ranging networks, the group was unable to build fruitful coalitions elsewhere.[56]

Secondly, feminism allowed them to synthesise the work of Erving Goffman and Louderback within an understanding of oppression and resistance as everyday experience.[57] Although they recognised social forces at play, they were aware that fat oppression took place in the prosaic spaces of ordinary life and affected women in particular ways.

Thirdly, the group established an analysis of fat oppression based on gender and radical lesbian identity.[58] Greta Rensenbrink points

53 Mayer, "Foreword."
54 Judy Freespirit and Aldebaran, *Fat Liberation Manifesto*, Largesse Fat Liberation Archives. Edited by The Fat Underground (Los Angeles/New Haven, CT: The Fat Underground/Largesse Fat Liberation Archives, 1973).
55 Fishman, "Life in the Fat Underground".
56 Aldebaran, "1974 Letter from Aldebaran to Karen Jones."
57 Goffman, *Stigma*; Louderback, *Fat Power*; Fishman, "Life in the Fat Underground".
58 Fat feminist analyses such as these could not have existed without The Fat

out that The Fat Underground regarded fat hatred as a component of patriarchy, "The intensity of women's fear of fat was fundamental to women's oppression, The Fat Underground theorised".[59] As a result of this they did not look to men as agents of their liberation.

We saw ourselves as, um, lawless.

Charlotte: You didn't ask for anybody's permission.

No, that was the whole point of feminism, right!

Charlotte: Right right right!

[laughs] Up until then we had to ask somebody, some male person, usually. And as feminists we got to make our own decisions, and were just running with it, and it was SO FREEING. (Judy)

Fourthly, The Fat Underground was a collective that sought to question power. Although some members' actions were significant or memorable, it was a group without formal leadership where decisions were made together. The Fat Underground maintained an unstructured membership. Archivist Karen Stimson lists 19 members but these are difficult to verify because people came and went, and the group was associated with overlapping organisations including The Radical Feminist Therapy Collective, The Fat Women's Problem-Solving Group, and other consciousness-raising groups that The Fat Underground convened.[60]

Underground. Laurie Ann Lepoff et al, "The Fats of Life: Reflections on the Tyranny of Fatophobia," *Off Our Backs* 13, no. 3 (1983): 30-32; Elizabeth A. Edwards, "Letter: Weight Oppression," *Off Our Backs* 19, no. 8 (1989): 26; Kathy Freeperson, "Letter: Heavy Punishment," *Off Our Backs* 13, no. 5 (1983): 30.
59 Greta Rensenbrink, "Fat's No Four-Letter Word: Fat Feminism and Identity Politics in the 1970s and 1980s" in *Historicizing Fat in Anglo-American Culture*, edited by Elena Levy-Navarro, 213-43 (Columbus, OH: The Ohio State University Press, 2010).
60 Karen Stimson, *The Fat Underground: The Original Radical Fat Feminists - a Commemorative Sourcebook from the Archives of Largesse, the Network for Size Esteem*

According to my interview with Judy, group members also lied about the number of people involved as an attention-grabbing strategy. Aldebaran acknowledged that the group maintained ambiguous boundaries:

> The Fat Underground is going through some profound structural changes right now, and I'm not even sure who's part of it and whether we're still a collective.[61]

The relative chaos of their organising brought some limitations and challenges. In 1974, for example, Aldebaran was afraid the group would founder because of a lack of leadership, though reassured herself of the benefits of non-hierarchical organising:

> I'm sitting here at my typewriter feeling like an old general. Isn't that absurd? No-one's talking about retiring! We are leader-full, not leader-less. (I hope, hope, hope. Now it's wait and see, work reasonably hard and have faith).[62]

Aldebaran's sense of responsibility and anxiety that nobody else would volunteer for duty hints that The Fat Underground's collective process was typically fraught. Yet with nobody officially in charge, a manifesto but no constitution or membership rules, people involved with the organisation were encouraged to take responsibility for its progression. This resulted in a dynamic space where fat feminists were able to reflect and act together, and this produced some of the most vigorous fat activism of the movement to date.

The Fat Underground offered a more sophisticated analysis of being fat than their contemporaries in fat activism, who tended to orient themselves towards NAAFA. Marvin Grosswirth's *Fat Pride* fails to connect fat oppression to wider social structures, or ally it with

(New Haven, CT: Largesse, 1995).
61   Aldebaran, "1974 Letter from Aldebaran to Karen Jones."
62   Aldebaran, "1974 Letter from Aldebaran to Karen Jones."

other liberation movements; it is presented simply as an unfortunate personal experience that can be remedied by fat-friendly consumerism and services.[63] In the timidly titled *Fat Can Be Beautiful,* Abraham I. Friedman, a normatively-sized obesity doctor, appropriates the terms of early fat liberation, describing NAAFA as a "militant" organisation, but ultimately advocates a model of weight loss and speaks of fatness in the usual abjecting manner.[64] Within feminism, Aldebaran mentions an unnamed group in New York who allied fat oppression with "lookism" but failed to provide an account of it within medicalisation or moral discourse.[65] This perhaps foreshadowed the feminist proxies for fat activism that came later.

Strategies

The Fat Underground manifested their political beliefs through several key activist strategies built around consciousness-raising and spectacle. Vivian F. Mayer refers to activities including "weekly drop-in rap groups for women." Like Fishman she mentions that retreats were held. Dana was associated with The Fat Underground and recalls activities such as eating together, and swimming.[66] The women undertook consciousness-raising through research. Mabel-Lois taught Aldebaran how to use medical libraries where they radically reappraised obesity research to publish a series of position papers on eating, health, job discrimination, psychiatry and sexism.[67] Their research

---

63 Marvin Grosswirth, *Fat Pride: A Survival Handbook* (New York: Jarrow Press, 1971).

64 Abraham I. Friedman, *Fat Can Be Beautiful: Stop Dieting, Start Living* (Berekeley, CA: Berekeley Publishing Corporation, 1974).

65 Aldebaran, "1974 Letter from Aldebaran to Karen Jones."

66 Mayer, "Foreword"; Fishman, "Life in the Fat Underground".

67 The Fat Underground, *Position Paper: Eating,* Largesse Fat Liberation Archive, Edited by The Fat Underground (Los Angeles/ New Haven CT: The Fat Underground/ Largesse Fat Liberation Archives, 1974); The Fat Underground, *Position Paper: Health of Fat Women...The Real Problem,* Largesse Fat Liberation Archives, Edited by The Fat Underground (Los Angeles/New Haven, CT: The Fat Underground/Largesse Fat Liberation Archives, 1974); *Position Paper: Job Discrimination; Position Paper:*

enabled fat activists to critique medicalised obesity discourse in the language of its advocates. In 1975 their involvement with the Women's Studies department at California State University led to them providing evidence against amphetamine prescription for weight loss before the California State Board of Medical Quality Assurance. Alongside their own publications, there is evidence of publishing elsewhere in *Sister* and *The Lesbian Tide*, Los Angeles women's liberation papers of the period, as well as Radical Therapy journals.[68] The group produced a video depicting them speaking to camera and outlining their beliefs about fat, as well as short sketches and conversations.[69]

More significantly, the group championed direct action and performance, promoting an ideal that was disobedient, unapologetic and anti-assimilationist.[70] This is illustrated by Judy who recalls a moment in The Fat Underground's video where Lynn Mabel-Lois delivers an attack on fat hatred directly to the camera.

> And she said: "I feel like a freak and I'm getting PROUD." She lifted her arm that was sleeveless and [shakes fat arm]. (Judy)

Psychiatry; Position Paper: Sexism.
68 Aldebaran, "We Are Not Our Enemies," *Sister,* December (1973): 6; Aldebaran, "Fat Liberation," *Issues in Radical Therapy* 3, no. Summer (1973); The Fat Underground, "More Women Are on Diets Than in Jail," *Sister,* November (1974): 4; Sharon Bas Hannah, "Naomi Cohen Choked on the Culture," *Sister,* September: 1; Lynn Mabel-Lois, "Fat Dykes Don't Make It," *Lesbian Tide* 4, no. 3 (1974): 11.
69 The Fat Underground, *The Fat Underground,* n.d. Video.
70 Theirs was a feminist analysis but it also harked back to the radical prankishness of the Fat-In. Judging by the books that Mayer lodged at the University of Connecticut's archives, she was heavily influenced by revolutionary culture of the period, as well as environmental activism. Jerry Rubin, *Do It! Scenarios of the Revolution* (New York: Simon and Schuster, 1970); Abbie Hoffman, *Revolution for the Hell of It* (New York: Dial Press, 1970); Alicia Bay Laurel, *Living on the Earth* (New York: Vintage Books, Random House, 1971); Saul D. Alinsky, *Rules for Radicals. A Practical Primer from Realistic Radicals* (New York: Vintage Books, 1972); Hugh Nash, ed. *Progress as If Survival Mattered. A Handbook for a Conserver Society* (San Francisco: Friends of the Earth, 1977).

The Fat Underground's most well-known action was at Women's Equality Day in Los Angeles in August 1974. The singer Mama Cass Elliot had died the month before. Media reports had turned her death into a punch-line, alleging she had choked to death on a ham sandwich.[71] But The Fat Underground theorised that Elliot's heart attack could have been aggravated by dieting. Mabel-Lois led a eulogy to the singer Cass Elliot whilst other group members performed a symbolic funeral procession with raised fists. Mabel-Lois accused the medical establishment of killing fat women, including Elliot, with weight loss.[72] The Fat Underground made use of zaps, a strategy of turning up where they were not wanted, pioneered in the peace movement and developed by the early gay rights activism.[73] They attended and disrupted a medical research conference and a TV channel promoting weight loss.[74]

Struggles

The Fat Underground were symbolically important as fearless freedom-fighters, originators, trail-blazers, but their struggles reveal the shortcomings of the myth. Despite their popularity in the Los Angeles women's scene, the group grappled with the effects of external and internal isolation and despondence. In 1974 they tried to establish more fat feminist consciousness-raising groups but were met with women who did not understand their mission and "were looking for the radical feminist way to be forever slim".[75] The assumption that lesbian

71 A rumour that circulated after the first physician's post mortem report, later found to be untrue. Eddi Fiegel, *Dream a Little Dream of Me: The Life of 'Mama' Cass Elliot.* (London: Pan, 2006).

72 Judy Freespirit and Aldebaran, "Writings from the Fat Underground" in *Shadow on a Tightrope: Writings by Women on Fat Oppression*, edited by Lisa Schoenfielder and Barb Wieser, 52-57 (Iowa City: Aunt Lute, 1983); Aldebaran, "1974 Letter from Aldebaran to Karen Jones"; Fishman, "Life in the Fat Underground".

73 Tommi Avicolli Mecca, *Smash the Church, Smash the State! The Early Years of Gay Liberation* (San Francisco: City Lights Books, 2008).

74 Mayer, "Foreword"; Fishman, "Life in the Fat Underground".

75 Aldebaran, "1974 Letter from Aldebaran to Karen Jones." Later *Fat Is A Feminist*

feminist community is open to fat women did not play out.[76] Private correspondence and papers produced by Aldebaran and Judy Freespirit from the early 1970s, archived by Karen Stimson through Largesse, reveal loneliness, longing and anxiety.[77] Freespirit's personal journals of the period present an ambivalent relationship to her fatness and lesbian sexuality, intensified by other problems. The group's founding members all experienced burn-out in the later stages.[78] Dana, who was encouraged by Freespirit to attend The Fat Women's Problem-Solving Group at The Women's Centre, and was later a member of The Fat Underground, remembers the more painful aspects of being fat that were present in the group:

> I recall many of the women in The Fat Women's Problem Solving Group had been on extensive, excessive reducing diets before coming to our meetings. Some of the women had serious physical problems due to diets and the resulting problems that result from being deprived of food. I also recall the immense emotional suffering of some of the women in the group. As a result of dieting and social stigma, women who were overweight and healthy and could have had the opportunity to live our lives in an atmosphere of acceptance of diversity, now often had eating issues, feelings of social rejection and physical problems, due to fat prejudice. Thus began our desire to take some action to make things right and to end fat prejudice. (Dana)

Dana reveals some of the internal tensions of the group concerning method, recalling that she experienced disapproval from some members

Issue was able to capitalise on this attitude.

76 Karen Heffernan, "Lesbians and the Internalization of Societal Standards of Weight and Appearance," *Journal of Lesbian Studies* 3, no. 4 (1999): 121-27; Aldebaran, "Letter: Liberal on Fat," *Off Our Backs* 10, no. 3 (1980): 31.

77 Stimson, *The Fat Underground: The Original Radical Fat Feminists - a Commemorative Sourcebook from the Archives of Largesse, the Network for Size Esteem.*

78 Mayer, "Foreword."

when she decided to prioritise her art and dance practice above her involvement with the group.

By 1976 The Fat Underground had ended acrimoniously, Freespirit had left the group, and there were problems with sexual and interpersonal relationships.[79] Mayer's claims that there were disagreements within the lesbian community on the West Coast about political correctness are corroborated by Yolanda Retter, who cites criticisms levied against the Radical Feminist Therapy Collective for its alleged abuse of power.[80]

Legacies

As early as 1974, Aldebaran recognised that the fat feminism she helped establish was a discourse that travelled through particular feminist networks.

> Through laying out the line on fat women and working with fat women at the weekly drop-in groups that we conduct, and through our presence at other movement actions and our friendship with other movement women, we have spread the idea.[81]

Despite their own struggles, ridicule, disbelief, resentment and silencing from political activists and other feminists, the ideas that the group founded continued beyond its demise, and even beyond death.[82]

79 In sharing these details I am reminded that historicising feminist social movements is a process of encountering trauma and high emotion. Deborah M. Withers, "Women's Liberation, Relationships and the 'Vicinity of Trauma,'" *Oral History*, no. 40, 1, Spring (2012): 79-88.
80 Mayer, "Foreword"; Susanna J. Sturgis, "Is This the New Thing We're Going to Have to Be P.C. About?" *Sinister Wisdom* 28 (1985): 16-47; Retter, "Lesbian Activism in Los Angeles, 1970-1979."
81 Aldebaran, "1974 Letter from Aldebaran to Karen Jones."
82 Core member Reanne Fagan died from breast cancer in November 1983. Stimson, "Fat Feminist Herstory, 1969-1993: A Personal Memoir".

This is exemplified through Ashley's account of stumbling across the canonical fat feminist text many years later in a setting far removed from the book's origins.

> I remember getting a copy of *Shadow On A Tightrope* from a Bradford charity shop.
>
> Charlotte: [gasps] WOWIE!
>
> Yes, isn't it! It must have been, I had a boyfriend up there so I think I was only about 17 or something, and it being this like, you know, I think at the time I wasn't really ready for it so it was a bit crazy and I shoved it at the bottom of my bookshelf and forgot about it and then came back to it when I was at university proper. Yeah, I sort of like that I'd come at it from that more haphazard scurrying, sort of scavenger way of contacting.
>
> Charlotte: I love that idea of the fatty scavenger, that's so beautiful, and it makes me–
>
> I think it really works with, like, the internet generation as well because I think there are so many people nowadays, they just come on to things entirely randomly and it's just, you know, like, just a link from a link from a link, and yeah I really think it works as much with that generation as much as it works with, you know, me finding this knackered book in a bookshop. (Ashley)

The Fat Underground broke up but fat feminist activism did not stop. Ashley's anecdote shows that it continues to pop up in unexpected places. I too was intrigued by how ideas that were generated in 1967 in New York travelled to me via Los Angeles. Aberystwyth in 1989 was a pretty remote place to be! Fat feminism is a place from which other things emerged so how did those ideas continue to move? How did and do I contribute to their movement? Perhaps these travels could also be understood as activism, indeed the word movement implied a phenomenon that is not static but dynamic, socially constructed, formed and maintained through people's actions. In the next chapter I will explore some of these travels, across space, time and culture. This is not the end of the story of fat feminism.

TRAVELLING

Fat activism does not stay still, it moves. This chapter is about how fat feminism travelled. Not only from Los Angeles to Aberystwyth, or from Iowa to Bradford, but through other threads and streams. I have found Kathy Davis' study useful as an example of how the feminist text *Our Bodies, Ourselves* formed a travelling feminist epistemology.[1] By this she means: "How feminist knowledge and knowledge practices move from place to place and are 'translated' in different cultural locations".[2] Davis writes about a feminist project that emerged out of a similar North American feminism to fat feminism, and there are direct connections to *Our Bodies, Ourselves* in this study. Like Davis, I use archival evidence, supported by accounts from the sample, to build a picture of the practical ways through which epistemology travelled, describing small acts and their cumulative effect over time and place. She regards this travelling feminism in quite abstract ways, but here it is more solid; it is what social change looks like. What follows is a loose chronology of fat feminist travels across country, through culture, across national borders and through queer space.

Davis' work is a product of anti-colonial scholarship developed by authors including Edward Said, Gayatri Chakravorty Spivak and Caren

1 Kathy Davis, *The Making of Our Bodies, Ourselves: How Feminism Travels Across Borders* (Durham, NC and London: Duke University Press, 2007).
2 Davis, *The Making of Our Bodies Ourselves*, 10. In case you have forgotten the earlier definition, epistemology is a way of saying 'ideas about how people come to know things'.

Kaplan.³ Their contributions stress the importance of remembering that travel is infused with power and abuse. I will address some of this later in this chapter by exploring how the notion of fat activism as a product of the US affects its transmission to the rest of the world. Power relationships within travelling fat feminist activism manifest through imperialism, xenophobia and racism. Here the US is the undisputed norm and the centre of all fat activism. Others are measured and measure themselves against this norm. It is part of a system of white and Western domination of the world.

MOVING WEST TO EAST THROUGH COMMUNITY

Greta Rensenbrink explains how early fat feminism was able to travel first from Los Angeles to the San Francisco Bay Area.⁴ The author explains that a cultural feminist infrastructure already existed in San Francisco by the mid 1970s, with a plethora of services, groups and meeting spaces, as well as communal houses. She writes that in 1975 a woman at The San Francisco Women's Centre started a consciousness-raising group for fat women, which spawned a group for fat lesbians and one for older fat women. Members of The Fat Underground visited these groups and further politicised their members. In 1978 or 1979, according to Rensenbrink, a Fat Underground lecture encouraged women to write and present their own fat manifestos at the Artemis feminist café. Around the same time a group called Life In The Fat Lane was founded. They were concerned with fighting fat oppression and consisted of members of the consciousness-raising group and The Gorgons, lesbian separatists,

3 Edward W. Said, *Orientalism* (New York: Pantheon Books, 1978); Edward W. Said, *The World, the Text, and the Critic* (Cambridge, MA: Harvard University Press, 1983); Gayatri Chakravorty Spivak, *In Other Worlds: Essays in Cultural Politics* (New York: Routledge, 1987); Caren Kaplan, *Questions of Travel: Postmodern Discourses of Displacement* (Durham, NC: Duke University Press, 1996).
4 Rensenbrink, "Fat's No Four-Letter Word: Fat Feminism and Identity Politics in the 1970s and 1980s."

who had been inspired by Fat Underground publications. Other groups appeared. Along with Lynn Ellen Marcus, Hannah Bannan, Martha Courtot, Leah Kushner and Barbara Penny, Judy Freespirit established Fat Chance Dance Troupe in Sonoma County, Northern California before settling in Oakland. In 1981 she started Fat Lip Reader's Theatre, a fat feminist writing and performance collective, which later produced a video, *Nothing to Lose*.[5] Diverse fat feminist culture in the Bay Area was able to flourish in the decade after The Fat Underground came to town because the conditions were ripe: there was already a welcoming community, primarily lesbian, that had access to particular resources. Fat lesbian feminists were able to support readings, exhibitions, more than one performance group, clothing swaps, a fat swim at Richmond Plunge, the Robust and Rowdy dances, Oakland's We Dance classes, the Let It All Hang Out block parties at Pride, and Cynthia Riggs' Making It Big clothes shop, to name a few interventions.[6]

New England was another important centre for fat feminism at that time, largely because of the organising undertaken by Judith Stein and her partner Meridith Lawrence, and the activities of the New Haven Fat Liberation Front, who were already part of The Fat Underground's network.

In 1978 or 1979 Stein founded a fat feminist group in the Boston area called, variously, Boston Fat Liberation, Boston Area Fat Liberation, Boston Area Fat Feminist Liberation and Boston Area Fat Lesbians (BAFL). The group met for discussion, support, and also Fatluck potluck dinner gatherings. When Stein left the group Lawrence co-organised it at the Cambridge Women's Centre. Verity attended this later group and fondly recalled the awkward earnestness of the meetings:

5 Fat Lip Reader's Theatre, *Nothing to Lose [Video]*. Oakland, CA: Wolfe Video, 1989. Video.
6 The photographer Cathy Cade, whose background was in anti-racist activism, the women's liberation movement and lesbian community, documented some of the fat activists and events of that period. Cathy Cade, *A Lesbian Photo Album: The Lives of Seven Lesbian Feminists* (Oakland, CA: Waterwoman Books, 1987).

So I'm picturing sitting in a room in a circle, there would be a topic and then they would start trying to get a conversation going and, you know, [Verity and Charlotte laugh] it wasn't always easy! (Verity)

With a growing support base, more ambitious gatherings took place. In April 1980 two meetings were convened over three days: The Feminist Fat Activist's Working Meeting and The New Haven Fat Women's Health Conference. These were organised by BAFL and The New Haven Fat Liberation Front, a short-lived group formed in 1976 consisting of Karen Scott-Jones (later Karen Stimson) and her then husband Darryl Scott-Jones as well as ex-Fat Underground members Aldebaran and Sharon Bas Hannah.[7] Scott-Jones had written about fat feminism for the National Organisation of Women and was part of NAAFA's Fat Feminist Caucus.[8] The April gatherings produced documentation and Fat Activists Together (F.A.T.) which, according to Stimson, was the first coalition of fat feminists, who went on to help publish *Shadow On A Tightrope* and circulated newsletters until 1982.[9]

Stein continued to publish a number of articles on fat and Jewish feminism, and wrote and circulated an information sheet about fat liberation at the Jewish Feminist Conference in San Francisco in 1982, according to Dykewomon's essay, "Travelling Fat."[10] A feminist health

7 The New York Times, "Fat Times in New Haven," http://www.eskimo.com/~largesse/Archives/NYT.html.

8 Stimson, "Fat Feminist Herstory, 1969-1993: A Personal Memoir".

9 Judith Stein, *Fat Oppression and Fat Liberation: Some Basic Ideas* (Boston, 1980); Schoenfielder and Wieser, *Shadow on a Tightrope*; Stimson, "Fat Feminist Herstory, 1969-1993: A Personal Memoir".

10 Judith Stein, *The New Haven Fat Women's Health Conference: Proceedings of the First Feminist Fat Activists' Working Meeting* (New Haven, CT: Fat Liberator Publications, 1980), Largesse Fat Liberation Archives; Judith Stein et al, "The Political History of Fat Liberation: An Interview," *The Second Wave* 3 (1981): 32-37; Judith Stein, "Fat Liberation: No Losers Here," *Sojourner* 6, no. 9 (1981): 8; Judith Stein, "On Getting Strong: Notes from a Fat Woman, in Two Parts" in *Shadow on a Tightrope: Writings by Women on Fat Oppression*, edited by Lisa Schoenfielder and Barb Wieser, 106-110 (Iowa City: Aunt Lute, 1983); Judith Stein, "Get Your Foot Off My Neck: Fat Liberation," *Gay*

worker, Stein advised the editorial collective for *Our Bodies, Ourselves*
and ensured that fat feminism was included in several US editions of
the book.[11] In 1984 and 1985 Stein and Lawrence presented fat feminist
radio shows on local radio for International Women's Day.[12] This work
enabled them to reach larger audiences for fat feminism and develop
alliances with Jewish feminist activism, the women's health communities
surrounding *Our Bodies, Ourselves*, as described by Davis, and in higher
education institutions.

Fat feminism was able to travel across the US because of national
kinship networks of the type described by Verity:

> Judith Stein and Judy Freespirit, they started talking on the phone,
> they corresponded, they maintained those relationships, and the
> thing about The Fat Underground is that they would send out
> newsletters and they advertised in the back of feminist periodicals,
> and so then, you know, like Elana [Dykewomon] read them in
> Northampton, and kept them under her bed, so you know it was like
> that. So there were groups that were trying to get the word out, you
> know, but you had to be in the world to find out about it. (Verity)

Fat feminist activism travelled through acts of friendship, circulating
small-run newsletters, buying cheap advertising in sympathetic
community periodicals, and preserving ad hoc archives. Mabel-Lois'
practical suggestion that, faced with fatphobia in lesbian communities, fat
feminist lesbians turn to each other for sexual and romantic partnerships,
helped create a somewhat insular miniature universe of overlapping

Community News, 28 June 1986, 6; Elana Dykewomon, "Travelling Fat" in *Shadow on
a Tightrope: Writings by Women on Fat Oppression*, edited by Lisa Schoenfielder and
Barb Wieser, 144-54 (Iowa City: Aunt Lute, 1983).

11 Boston Womens Health Collective, *The New Our Bodies, Ourselves* (New York:
Simon & Schuster, 1984).

12 Judith Stein and Meridith Lawrence, *Plain Talk About Fat [Radio]*, Boston:
Massachusetts Institute of Technology, 1984; Judith Stein and Meridith Lawrence, *30
Big Minutes with Fat Liberation [Radio]*, Boston: Massachusetts Institute of Technology,
1985.

friends and lovers who worked together as activists.[13] These were in-group activities, unavailable to outsiders who did not already know the codes of entry, which perhaps explains why this work remains obscured from broader discussion in Fat Studies and elsewhere. Nevertheless, the connections that facilitated this travelling fat feminist activism endure and are not locked into the past, but continue through networks of older fat feminists. Three of the people I interviewed, who met through one of the groups mentioned above, have remained in contact with each other for close to three decades.

CULTURAL JOURNEYS

Some of the methods of fat feminist cultural production enabled these kinship networks to thrive. These included consciousness-raising, independent publishing and mainstream media exposure, which resulted in the formation of a number of fat feminist activist groups.

Stein continued to develop fat feminism through a presence, including workshops and discussions, at the Michigan Womyn's Music Festival which was a major annual international gathering for radical feminists. Liat remarked that in 1979:

> ReaRae Sears is a white woman but she owns a tipi, and [Sears and Stein] brought the tipi and it became the meeting place for fat liberation. And so the first fat liberation meeting that I went to there, and I'm not sure it was the very first one, but the first one I attended, there must have been 50-75 women in a circle with Judith and ReaRae at the tipi, [...] standing up talking. (Liat)

From Michigan, according to a contributor to *A Queer and Trans Fat Activist Timeline*, and corroborated by Martha and Liat, other lesbian and fat activists in the Midwest began to adopt fat feminism, which culminated

13 Mabel-Lois, "Fat Dykes Don't Make It."

in the publication of *Shadow on a Tightrope: Writings by Women on Fat Oppression* in Iowa.[14] The collection of first person essays and accounts of fat feminism was originally mooted by The Fat Underground, with Aldebaran and Sharon Bas Hannah, who gave the book its title, trying and failing to publish it during their stay in New Haven. In 1978 Mayer began to sell packets of articles from the book's original manuscript as well as other articles and t-shirts through advertisements in feminist periodicals under the name *Fat Liberator Publications*. Liat was given the papers in 1978 by a housemate who had ordered them from a lesbian magazine. She remembered:

> Yeah it came from a woman who lived in LA who had been doing radical therapy stuff and she, I was living in [Michigan] in a group house, and there was a woman there [...] and we were living in this house together and she pulled out this bunch–, and it was I remember they, I think I still have it actually, it was all different colours, stapled, and she was like: "I think you might be interested in this," I read it and I was like, SNAP, I mean it was just like a massive connection, light-bulbs going off, you know, and there I was. And I was, like, no turning back. (Liat)

In 1980 Mayer stopped doing fat activism. She handed *Fat Liberator Publications* to Diane Denne, who then passed them on to Lisa Schoenfielder and Barb Wieser. The pair advertised in radical feminist periodicals for new contributions for the book, which they published alongside older Fat Underground material as *Shadow on a Tightrope*. The book made quite a splash in the feminist press of the time, it was crucial to the development of fat activism as a national and transnational affair, and it remains an important document of early fat feminism and the theorising of fat oppression.[15]

14 Schoenfielder and Wieser, *Shadow on a Tightrope: Writings by Women on Fat Oppression*.
15 Loraine Hutchins, "Review: Shadow on a Tightrope: Writings by Women on Fat Oppression by Lisa Schoenfielder and Barb Wieser," *Off Our Backs* 15, no. 3 (1985):

North America, and other Western locations including the UK, to some extent, enjoyed a rich culture of local and national lesbian feminist periodicals that peaked in volume in the 1970s and 1980s and then petered out. It was through these publishing networks that fat feminism travelled. Susan Koppelman acknowledges that the proliferation of fat feminist publishing in periodicals such as *Sister, Lesbian Contradiction* and *Plexus,* became a home for a fat feminist activist "bravura literature".[16] Some journals devoted special issues or sections to fat, for example *Matrix* and *Common Lives/Lesbian Lives.*[17] Other journals had sympathetic editors, for example Elana Dykewomon at *Sinister Wisdom,* who were themselves involved with fat activism.[18] Verity was part of this publishing scene and explained how editorial policies encouraging fat feminist writing engendered confidence and security in her, knowing there was somewhere she could share her work and that journal editors and readers would take her seriously:

> Well I guess the other thing, you know, that I was thinking about having looked at that huge pile of [lesbian journals, Verity had recently shown me her collection] like so, and Elana, she wasn't the editor of *Sinister Wisdom* when I first got published there, but she was the editor of *Sinister Wisdom* for many years and that was a place where I could be reliably published. Right now I don't have that, but I knew if I sent something out it would be very seriously

24-25; Rita Stockwell, "Letter: Shadow-Boxing," *Off Our Backs* no. 8: 34; Loraine Hutchins, "Letter: And Response," *Off Our Backs* no. 8: 34; Ruth Millar, "A Review of Shadow on a Tightrope: Writings by Woman on Fat Oppression, Edited by Lisa Schoenfielder & Barb Wieser, Aunt Lute Book Company, U.S.A., 1983, Available in the U.K. At £6.95," *Gossip: A Journal of Lesbian Feminist Ethics* 4 (1987): 44-50.
16 Koppelman, *The Strange History of Suzanne Lafleshe (and Other Stories of Women and Fatness).*
17 Matrix, *Embracing Our Beauty, Claiming Our Space: Voices of Fat Liberation* (Santa Cruz, CA: Matrix, 1987); Leslie Baker, "Meridith and Judith," *Common Lives/Lesbian Lives* 12 (1984): 27.
18 Judy Freespirit, "Doing Donahue," *Common Lives/Lesbian Lives* 20 (1986): 5-14; Susan Stinson, "Whole Cloth," *Common Lives/Lesbian Lives* 19 (1986) : 58-61; Susan Stinson, "Belly Song," *Sinister Wisdom* 32 (1987): 111-13.

considered and it might well be taken, and fat was no barrier, and so I sent and sent and sent and I would write and I would send and I knew, you know, that there was a place. (Verity)

Publication conferred legitimacy to the seemingly absurd project of fat activism. Lesbian feminist periodicals were an important site for fat feminism and no doubt contributed to its spread, but their ephemeral nature was no match for a book-length work such as *Shadow On A Tightrope*. Verity, again, explained that the book was important because it represented a community that had been experienced until then as nebulous and isolated:

> There was a sense of connection to a larger movement in that way but it wasn't based in geography. I don't know of other fat groups that were active in the area. But then we read *Shadow On A Tightrope*, it seemed that there were people in other places. (Verity)

The combination of networks of fat feminists produced through the Michigan Womyn's Music Festival, and through the abundance of feminist publishing activity, together with the feeling that "there were people in other places" exploded into apparent material reality during the period that *Shadow On A Tightrope* was first published. Fat feminism enjoyed mainstream national exposure in the US with Fat Lip's appearance on *The Phil Donahue Show*, and through *Radiance* magazine, established in 1984.[19] The Fat Avengers, a lesbian separatist fat feminist group based in Seattle, produced a calendar, *Images of Our Flesh*, in 1983, featuring photographs by Cookie Andrews-Hunt.[20] Jenny Ellison found evidence of at least 15 fat activist groups in Canada between 1979 and 2000.[21] Elana

19 Freespirit, "Doing Donahue." Radiance was published quarterly by Alice Ansfield in Oakland until 2000.

20 Cookie Andrews-Hunt, *Images of Our Flesh* (Seattle: The Fat Avengers, 1983).

21 Ellison, "Weighing In: The 'Evidence of Experience' and Canadian Fat Women's Activism."

Dykewomon indicates that there were other lesbian feminist fat liberation organisations across the US, including Fat Is A Lesbian Issue in New York, and The Lesbian Fat Activists Network in Woodstock; Lesbians of Size in Portland and Sisters of Size in Seattle; Big, Beautiful Lesbians in Washington DC; Sisters Are Fighting Fat Oppression in Minneapolis; and groups unnamed by her in Atlanta, Boston, Northampton Massachusetts, Canada, the UK, Australia and The Netherlands, where Vet Vrieg sprung from a fat feminist gathering in Amsterdam in 1980.[22]

Yet this upsurge of activity was coupled with a sense of unreality, the product of a lack of documentation and communication between groups.

> No one knows how many fat liberation struggles took place in the last decade. We have lacked a way to communicate with each other. Under the triple stresses of fat oppression, isolation, and the disinterest or even hostility with which our pleas for support were often met, fat activists have all too often taken the frustrations out on each other and destroyed our own organisations before they could take root. For years, I have heard rumours of fat women's groups in Baltimore, Philadelphia, elsewhere, that formed, then toppled into oblivion with no proof that they ever existed.[23]

Groups disappeared as quickly as they had arrived. Although they were the outcome of a travelling fat feminist activism, that alone could not sustain them in a context where they were already facing social marginalisation as fat people and lesbians in a period of feminist ideological conflict where burn-out was common.

---

22 Elana Dykewomon, "Fat Liberation" in *Encyclopedia of Lesbian and Gay Histories and Cultures, Volume 1*, edited by George Haggerty and Bonnie Zimmerman, 290-91 (New York: Garland Publishing, 2000).
23 Mayer, "Foreword."

TRANSNATIONAL CROSSINGS

Fat feminism travelled to the UK by the same means that it had travelled through the US: the existence of a strong feminist community that had already developed audiences and resources of its own, *Shadow On A Tightrope*, and kinship networks. Heather Smith, one of the founders of the London Fat Women's Group which was the first fat feminist activist group in the UK, explained how it was formed:

> A few years ago a friend of mine and I read a book on fat oppression[24] and what we thought was that we should try to write an article in the British feminist press to try and get it put on the political agenda here so that it would be seen as an issue that was worth, you know, considering. And once the article was published in a feminist magazine, from that we got lots of responses and this is how the group has grown and grown.[25]

The London Fat Women's Group began by publishing and promoting their ideas in the feminist press between 1986 and 1989.[26] Fat feminists in the UK had significant access to national media as relatively autonomous creators. Nancy Roberts, a feminist, broadcaster and founding member of Spare Tyre Theatre Company,[27] helped introduce anti-diet and fatshion

24 I am guessing that this book was *Shadow On A Tightrope*. A British edition was later published by Rotunda, a short-lived fat feminist publishing house. Rotunda Press, "Watchout Rotunda Is Coming!" *Spare Rib* no. 211 (1990): 54.

25 BBC, *Fat Women Here to Stay*, Open Space, edited by Community Programme Unit UK, 1989. Television.

26 Amanda Hayman, "Fat Oppression," *Gossip: A Journal of Lesbian Feminist Ethics* 3 (1986): 66-72; Jenkins and Smith, "Fat Liberation"; Linda Bean at al, "Body Consciousness," *Gossip: A Journal of Lesbian Feminist Ethics* 3 (1986): 20-21; Heather Smith, "Creating a Politics of Appearance," *Trouble + Strife* 16, no. Summer (1989): 36-41; Tina Jenkins and Margot Farnham, "As I Am," *Trouble + Strife* 13 (1988); Sue Teddern, "Fat Pride and Prejudice," *The Guardian*, 14 February 1989, 21; Vron, "Taking up Space: From Fat Oppression to Fat Liberation," *From the Flames* no. 4 (1991): 4-13.

27 See http://www.unfinishedhistories.com/history/companies/spare-tyre for more information on Spare Tyre.

discourse to the mainstream in her feel-good 1983 Thames Television talk show *Nancy At Large,* and its related publications.[28] Incidentally, Roberts' connections to Orbach through The Women's Therapy Centre, as well as fat feminism through The London Fat Women's Group, and her dual US-UK citizenship, characterises her as something of a hybrid figure in fat activism, transnationally traversing polarised discourse.

The London Fat Women's Group organised a conference on 11 February 1989.[29] By promoting the conference in the mainstream media, it became a high profile event and the group was not prepared for such a level of visibility. Smith writes that many women had to be turned away from the conference and that there were problems with intrusive newspaper reporters.[30] Despite numerous organisational hassles the conference was an important consciousness-raising event:

> For a few hours we stepped out of our isolation and into an unfamiliar reality. It felt like the alchemy of other fat women's energy collected and combined and strengthened us all in ways we are not used to. The world was different; it was exciting and emotional and scary. I know the way I felt for days afterwards was different from anything before or since: a brief glimpse of what it might feel like not to be oppressed.[31]

In her own report of the conference, Smith maintains a commitment to the broad anti-oppressive practice that had been initiated by The Fat Underground 15 years previously.[32] But the reaction to this activism within British feminism was mixed, with attacks launched on associates

28 Roberts, *Breaking All the Rules.*
29 "The conference aims to highlight the oppression that fat women suffer, and celebrate liberation from fawn crimplene tent dresses!!" Anonymous, "National Fat Women's Conference," *Spare Rib* no. 197 (1988): 89; London Fat Women's Group, "Fat Women's Conference." *Spare Rib* no. 193: 54.
30 Smith, "Creating a Politics of Appearance."
31 Vron, "Taking up Space."
32 Vron, "Taking up Space."

of The London Fat Women's Group by normatively-sized women, and critiques by other fat feminists.[33]

The London Fat Women's Group ended shortly after the conference and anecdotal evidence suggests that this was largely due to in-fighting relating to the television appearances, and burn-out.[34] Diana Pollard reported that, as in North America, local groups were formed after the conference, but she does not name them or elaborate this claim.[35]

This is where I became part of things. I watched the London Fat Women's Group's television appearances and wanted to be a part of fat feminism but, by the time I was in a position to participate, the group had ended. I tried to re-establish a Fat Women's Group in London a couple of years later. I followed the earlier group's strategy of placing an advert in Spare Rib, the most prominent British feminist magazine of the time, and a number of people responded.[36] Some members of the first group were supportive of this second group and wanted to participate, others could not be found. Varying numbers of fat women met monthly for approximately two years from 1992, but I was inexperienced, we lacked direction, failed to operate as a collective and, aside from producing a popular newsletter, the group foundered. I also burned-out and left in

33 Diana Pollard, "Beyond Fat Liberation: Towards a Celebration of Size Diversity" in *Sizeable Reflections: Big Women Living Full Lives*, edited by Shelley Bovey, 22-37 (London: The Women's Press, 2000); Hayman, "Fat Oppression"; Lynette Mitchell, "Skinny Lizzie Strikes Back: An Apologia for Thin Women's Liberation," *Gossip: A Journal of Lesbian Feminist Ethics* 3 (1986): 40-44.

34 Pollard, "Beyond Fat Liberation."

35 Pollard, "Beyond Fat Liberation." On the other hand, there is evidence of this in *Spare Rib* magazine: a call for participants, "FATSPIRIT will celebrate the joys and contributions of abundantly fat women, in words and images. FATSPIRIT will include writings and visuals by women of many different cultures, races and ancestries, representing how fat women see ourselves and each other, having fun, being loved and lovable, and loving being fat," which apparently sank without trace. Cathy and Zhana, "Fat Women Celebrate!" *Spare Rib* no. 216 (1990): 55; and a group in Manchester who seemed to fail for lack of funds and interest from the beginning. Fat Women's Group, "Fat Women's Group," *Spare Rib* no. 208 (1989): 88; Manchester Fat Women's Group, "Manchester Fat Women's Group," *Spare Rib* no. 203: 57.

36 Charlotte Cooper, "Political and Social Group for Other Fat Women," *Spare Rib* no. 233 (1992): 48.

1994 when Diana Pollard assumed its leadership. Under her, The Fat Women's Group produced an exhibition of fat women's art in 1995 at the London Women's Centre, which had been home to both Fat Women's Groups and the Fat Women's Conference. In 1996 Pollard re-launched The Fat Women's Group to include men, naming it SIZE: The National Size Acceptance Network. Through SIZE, Pollard authored *Freesize* magazine in 1998, but this failed to thrive.[37]

Thorny relationships between Pollard, Shelley Bovey, the publisher of my first book, and I echo the difficulties faced by members of The Fat Underground as that organisation fractured and ended. They also illustrate the role that in-fighting played in how fat feminist activism in the UK at that time came to be documented. In her account of that period of fat feminism, which was edited by Bovey and published through The Women's Press, Pollard omits all mention of my name and contributions to the movement though she knew about and benefitted from them. I have described how relationships and kinship networks helped establish and develop fat feminist activist discourse, and that in some cases they endured. But it is also worth noting that activist relationships can be fragile or volatile, that publishers' politics also raise the legitimacy of some voices over others, and this too affects a social movement's intergenerational documentation and transmission.[38] Where material evidence is already scarce and obscure, this writing-out of history further marginalises the contributions of fat feminist activists. Few people embroiled in these disputes are willing to speak publicly about them because of anger, shame and regret that can last for decades.

Meanwhile, fat activism in the UK was moving away from lesbian feminism, a radical critique of fat oppression, or fat liberation.[39] Bovey's

---

37 Diana Pollard, *Freesize*, Vol. 3, London, 1999.

38 Less controversially this writing-out can also happen when actions do not fit a pre-existing narrative. For example, in 1991 I was a runner-up in a modelling completion organised by *Pretty Big*, and in 1992 I helped launch a BBW club called *Planet Big Girl* with my friend Amanda Bailey. Both were formative for me regarding my fat activism but they seem at odds with the identity I am building of myself in this book as a queer activist who is a product of radical lesbian fat feminism.

39 Simic proposes that this shift was about embracing fat positive identity and

popular critical work on fat, which was partly researched at The London
Fat Women's Group conference, became more apologetic in later
editions, and culminated in her renouncement of fat liberation and the
publication, by the same radical feminist publisher that had handled my
own *Fat & Proud*, of a book explaining how to lose weight.[40] Mary Evans
Young established her franchise *Dietbreakers* through a campaigning
presence and shifted the discourse towards an anti-diet and early HAES
rhetoric that did not always include fat people.[41] She was not the only
entrepreneur to see the value of fat activism during this period, *Extra
Special*, *Yes!* and *Pretty Big* were three women's magazines which focused
on the plus size fashion industry and the bright and breezy self-help
approach to fat that had been popularised by Roberts. These magazines
developed a loyal readership and organised events such as modelling
competitions, awards ceremonies, holidays and get-togethers which
fostered community, business alliances and customer bases. This was
also happening in Europe with the formation of Allegro Fortissimo
in France in 1989, which had a similar focus on fashion though later
expanded to consumer rights and advocacy. Whilst the promotion of self-
acceptance through fat politics was good for business, the radical lesbian
feminism of the London Fat Women's Group and their predecessors
was alien to these far more mainstream projects. What originated as a
branch of a social movement allied with other liberation movements
was unable to leverage its legitimacy and longevity in the UK. Broader
radical community support was not forthcoming and there was less of
a supportive lesbian feminist infrastructure compared to the US. By
accepting mainstream media appearances, The London Fat Women's
Group were able to broadcast their ideas to a mass audience but it also
made them vulnerable. Their ideas became appropriated into a discourse

celebration but, as I will explain here, I disagree. Simic, "Fat as a Feminist Issue:
A History."

40 Bovey, *Being Fat Is Not a Sin*; Shelley Bovey, *The Forbidden Body: Why Being Fat Is
Not a Sin* (London: Pandora, 1994); Bovey, *What Have You Got to Lose?*

41 Mary Evans Young, *Diet Breaking: Having It All without Having to Diet* (London:
Hodder & Stoughton, 1995).

of marketing, celebrity and leadership, generic body politics, assimilation and consumerism.

QUEER TRANSMISSIONS

The origins of fat feminism are immersed within a feminism that is problematic, maligned, unfashionable and obscure, that is, radical lesbian feminism, including, at times, lesbian separatism. Critiques of this feminism surfaced within queer, third wave and postmodern feminisms because of, for example, its essentialism and its fundamentalism.[42] The lesbian sex wars, brutal fights about sex and patriarchy, and the emergence of queer gender politics and activism were similarly responsible for its loss of authority.[43] Radical lesbian feminist separatism is commonly constructed in opposition to third wave queer feminism.[44] But Kris remarked that they are closely related through DIY culture:

> Well I think in part it is because the third wave's roots come from lesbian separatism and so it's that. So there's that. The idea that if the world isn't going to be the way you want it to, fuck the world, make your own world. (Kris)

Judging by the kinds of articles that were appearing in the mainstream feminist press in the US by the late 1990s and early 2000s, fat feminist activism was also stalling and being overtaken by a body positive/body

42 Anonymous, "Queers Read This," http://www.qrd.org/qrd/misc/text/queers. read.this; Annamarie Jagose, *Queer Theory* (Melbourne: Melbourne University Press, 1996); Nikki Sullivan, *A Critical Introduction to Queer Theory* (Edinburgh: Edinburgh University Press, 2003); Iain Morland and Annabelle Willox, *Queer Theory* (Basingstoke: Palgrave Macmillan, 2005).

43 Gayle Rubin, "Thinking Sex: Notes for a Radical Theory of the Politics of Sexuality" in *Pleasure and Danger*, edited by Carole Vance, 267-319 (Boston: Routledge & Keegan Paul, 1984); Patrick Califia, *Public Sex: The Culture of Radical Sex*, 2nd ed. (San Francisco: Cleis Press, 2000).

44 Eve Kosofsky Sedgwick, *Epistemology of the Closet* (Berkeley and Los Angeles: University of California Press, 1990); Danielle Clarke, "Finding the Subject: Queering the Archive," *Feminist Theory* 5, no. 1 (2004): 79-83.

image discourse.[45] But changes and shifts in fat activist community suggest that there are continuities and that fat feminism continued to travel into less mainstream queer and third wave feminisms.

The Bay Area continued to be an important location for fat feminism and in 1994 a group of young activists published the first of six issues of the zine *FaT GiRL*. This project had close connections to earlier fat feminism, and at least one founding collective member, Max Airborne, had been introduced to fat activism by radical lesbian feminist separatists.[46] *FaT GiRL* established fat dyke identity but left that concept open to interpretation and inclusion of people who were beginning to organise around genderqueer and trans identities. At the same time, the zine published articles by and about earlier fat feminist activism, there was no explicit editorial divide between the older and newer radical fat lesbian and queer activism, it was inclusive. *FaT GiRL* continued to build fat feminist culture through publishing, working collectively, and engaging closely with identity politics, oppression and liberation.[47] As a queer publication it tolerated ambiguities and ambivalences and did not simply reproduce a body positive mind-set.[48] As with the fat feminism

45 I have been struck by the encroachment of feminist body image discourse as a proxy for fat feminism in the archives of the US journal *Off Our Backs*. The journal was criticised by fat feminists for ignoring fat activism and for reproducing fatphobia and represents a mainstream feminist media's unease in engaging with fat. Deb Roark, "Letter: Sized up &Boxed In," *Off Our Backs* 6, no. 5 (1976): 30; Aldebaran, "Letter: Oob Perpetuating Stereotypes," *Off Our Backs* 9, no. 11 (1979): 31; Elly Janesdaughter, "Letter: Fatophobic Feminists," *Off Our Backs* no. 7: 28 (1979); Aldebaran, "Letter: Liberal on Fat," *Off Our Backs* 10, no. 3 (1980): 31; Katy WildSister, "Letter: Not Buying It," *Off Our Backs* 20, no. 8 (1990): 34; debby Earthdaughter, "Letter: Diet Pills Next?" *Off Our Backs* 21, no. 3 (1991): 35; Theresa Elg, "Letter: Weight Ad Unacceptable," *Off Our Backs* 21, no. 5 (1991): 34. The 2004 special issue on body image, the journal's main engagement with fat, is bland in comparison to the early community voices represented on its letters page. Off Our Backs, *Off Our Backs: Body Image*, Vol. 34 (Arlington, VA: Off Our Backs, 2004). The discourse shifts to self-acceptance, stigma and eating cake. Later in this book I will talk about the gentrification of fat activism, and I would argue that the pages of *Off Our Backs* are a microcosm of this process.

46 Max Airborne, "True Tales from Life in the Fat Lane," *FaT GiRL* 3 (1995): 48.

47 A. Hernandez, "Judy Freespirit," *FaT GiRL* 1 (1994): 6-7; Barbara et al, "Fat Girl Roundtable 3: Racism and Fat Hatred," *FaT GiRL* 3 (1995): 42-47; Vale, "Fat Girl."

48 Lynne Gerber, "Movements of Luxurious Exuberence: Georges Bataille and

of the previous decade, *FaT GiRL* used DIY resources and networks, but these had changed by 1994 to encompass desktop publishing and online technologies. These enabled the zine to be published autonomously and relatively cheaply, to reach a large interactive readership, and to benefit from zine publishing and queercore (queer punk) networks rather than a lesbian journal distribution model or a mainstream publishing model such as that used by *Radiance*.[49]

Nevertheless, there were departures. Where fat dykes were depicted in less sexualised terms in other early feminist representations, for example in Andrews-Hunt's calendar, or in Leslie Baker's photo-spread for *Common Lives/Lesbian Lives* of Judith Stein and Meridith Lawrence at home together, *FaT GiRL* published explicit photographs. These images queered notions of lesbian sexuality and revelled in sexual diversity, especially SM, that would have been taboo in other feminisms.[50] These raw representations of fat queer sexuality and culture reflected the milieu from which the zine was produced. Elliot recalled an abundance of fat, queer, kinky sex at the time:

> So in the early '90s, you know, '93, '94, '95, many of us that were part of the group that started *FaT GiRL* were also part of the leather scene. [...] And so we were going to play parties and leather-related events. Um, there was a lot of fat people! A lot of fat people. Fat people fucking, fat people having sex, fat people being seen as hot. There was this little tiny subculture where we could see that, you know, [...] there was just a good number of fat people out there, publicly having sex. And radical sex. (Elliot)

Fat Politics" in *Negative Ecstasies: Georges Bataille and the Study of Religion*, edited by Jeremy Biles and Kent L. Brintnall, 19-37 (New York: Fordham University Press, 2015).
49 Devra Polack, "Queer Punks Chew the Fat," *FaT GiRL* 6 (1996): 6-7.
50 Andrews-Hunt, *Images of Our Flesh*; Baker, "Meridith and Judith"; Susan Johnson et al, "The Sa/Me Debate," *FaT GiRL* 4 (1995): 8-9; Betty Rose Dudley, "A Fat, Vulgar, Angry, Slut," *FaT GiRL* 4 (1995): 21-22.

FaT GiRL ended by the late 1990s but fat feminism continued to travel through other queer networks, such as Pretty Porky and Pissed Off, a performance-activist group based in Toronto.[51] Around that time fat feminism in the US found greater expression in one-off events: 1997's Fall Fat Women's Gathering in Seattle had been a great success, for example, and there had been a well-attended rally against fat hatred for the writer Susan Stinson in Northampton, Massachusetts in 2000.[52] In Portland, Oregon, Fat Girl Speaks, a series of events incorporating performance and workshops, carried on the work into the mid 2000s, and a consciousness-raising/ fat positive youth project called Phat Camp was also active at this time. In the UK this queer sensibility leaked through into the inaugural Miss Lesbian Beauty, organised by the fat femme Amy Lamé in 1997 and won by BJ, a fat dyke who listed her hobbies as "horse riding and bondage".[53]

NOLOSE was another intergenerational fat feminist space that traversed the alleged divide between lesbian and queer. NOLOSE was originally a false acronym for National Organisation for Lesbians of Size, but today it is used as a name in its own right. It was founded by Dot Nelson-Turnier in 1997. Nelson-Turnier had been a member of the various FLAB (Fat is a Lesbian Issue/Fat Lesbian Action Brigade) fat feminist groups based in New York, convened by Shira Stone and Gail Horowitz. Nelson-Turnier was inspired to act after reading fatphobic comments made about a fat cover model for the periodical *The Lesbian Connection*.[54] This typified the continuing problem of fatphobia in

51 Mitchell, "Pissed Off."
52 Susan Stinson, "Speakout against Fat Hatred," *Healthy Weight Journal* 14, no. 4 (2000): 62.
53 Philip Reay-Smith, "The World's First Lesbian Beauties," *The Pink Paper*, 4 July 1997. BJ was the guest of honour at *The Fat of the Land: A Queer Chub Harvest Festival*, of which more later, where she opened the event by cutting the ribbon with a flick-knife.
54 Dot Nelson-Turnier, "Why a National Organization for Lesbians of Size?" http://www.nolose.org/old/Newsletter/nolose01.html; Shira Stone, "Speaking out, Reaching Out," http://www.nolose.org/old/Newsletter/nolose04.html; Diana Lee, "In the Beginning... " http://www.nolose.org/old/Events/2000_Conference/conference_2000.html; Diana Lee, "Dot Nelson-Turnier: Nolose Woman for the New Millennium,"

lesbian communities where the lesbian media's support of fat feminism could not be assumed.[55] Nelson-Turnier initially wanted to establish a national network of local groups which, as Mayer had pointed out, needed better lines of communication.[56] Eventually NOLOSE became a series of conferences, beginning in 2000 in New York state. In 2001 the first board was formed by Dianne Rubinstein, Stone and Diana Lee. NOLOSE has continued since then, and has been held on the East Coast of the US, New England and, latterly, Oakland in California. It has supported smaller spin-off projects in New York like The Fat Girl Flea Market and Jiggle-O in 2003, as well as a zine and local gatherings.

In 2004 a new group of NOLOSE board members set about queering the organisation by developing long-running community discussions about the inclusion of all genders in a space that had previously been women-only, and addressing the intersectionality of fat politics.[57] There was a need to create a space where people of all genders could address fat because trans communities at that time could not be depended upon to be supportive of fat people. For example:

> I think that some of the specific ways that trans communities have felt like they, like they'll throw fat people under the bus, you know, is around, are around how very often that people who are female-bodied or transitioning, and sometimes through the process of whether they go up or not through the process of hormones and of taking T [testosterone], you know, sometimes they gain weight and there's a sense of fear around that, a very very real sense of fear around transmasculine communities, somehow

http://www.nolose.org/old/Newsletter/nolose10.html.

55 Mabel-Lois, "Fat Dykes Don't Make It"; Unsigned for obvious reasons, "Letter: Fat Kills," *Off Our Backs* 9, no. 7 (1979): 28; Mitchell, "Skinny Lizzie Strikes Back: An Apologia for Thin Women's Liberation"; Wilton, *Good for You: A Handbook of Lesbian Health and Wellbeing.*

56 Mayer, "Foreword"; Dot Nelson-Turnier, "Notes from the Founder," http://www.nolose.org/old/Newsletter/nolose02.html.

57 Tara Shuai et al, "Nolose Policy Change: Inclusion and Moving from Identity to Intention," http://www.nolose.org/11/genderpolicy.php.

that that's actually feminising, which is interesting, it's interesting that fat is seen as something that morphs you, you know, and morphs bodies. See to me that's exciting. (Paz)

A number of older lesbian feminist participants responded by withdrawing from the conference, their anxieties expressed here by Martha:

> I think the other thing that's changed that's been hard for me, and I still wrestle with is, as an old time lesbian feminist, dealing with gender, gender identity, transgender, the whole community has shifted to a place that's not altogether comfortable for me. So I'm sort of trying to think about well what does that mean, and what do you want to do with that, and that's been mostly an intellectual activity at this point. But I mean I think that's part of what kept us from NOLOSE in part for a while was, that's not how I identify my lesbian community, and it's like I think I'm at the point now where I can say, "Get over yourself and take what you can," you know, but it's different, it's different. (Martha)

In 2010 NOLOSE moved to Oakland, capitalising on its community of older fat lesbian feminists, and women like Martha began to return. But although NOLOSE community discussion about gender is an example of how a hybrid fat feminism can become established in the borderlands between different ideologies, this is not an easy process and is the subject of on-going argument. The struggle reflects continuing and perhaps unavoidable activist investment in agreement, sameness and unity, particularly within identity politics. At the same time, the existence of an organisation that reflects and serves diverse feminisms, including those that present relationships of seemingly intractable dissonance, suggests that many accounts are possible in particular sites.

I have left Bears out of this discussion of fat activism's queer travels. This is mainly because they tend to lack a feminist basis. Ron Suresha's Bear history both patronises and belittles fat feminism and Alex Robertson

Textor points out that the Big Men's Movement is not feminist, and is at times anti-feminist.[58] Jason Whitesel omits a feminist analysis of his research subjects.[59] Other accounts of Bear culture suggest that fat activist principles cannot be assumed. Laurence Brown, a normatively-sized man who fetishises fat Bears, argues that what makes fat men sexually appealing to him might be stigma and discrimination; and Lawrence D. Mass, a physician who is also active in Bear community in the US, criticises the cultural imperative for slenderness, yet also denounces NAAFA for encouraging self-acceptance in fat people.[60] Nathaniel Pyle and Michael Loewy deny that Bears are fat activists because they are conservative and groups such as Girth and Mirth are social, not political, as though conservatism and the social are not also political.[61] Brendan Gough and Gareth Flanders locate Bears within a social movement that celebrates fatness, yet the authors look to Bear culture as a site for weight loss interventions.[62]

Things may be changing, not least because queer masculinities are changing. Chris Vargas and Greg Youmans make art about trans Bear identity informed by fat feminism and fat activism.[63] I have enjoyed

58 Ron Suresha, "Bear Roots" in *The Bear Book: Readings in the History and Evolution of a Gay Male Subculture*, edited by Les K. Wright, 41-49 (New York: Harrington Park Press, 1997); Alex Robertson Textor, "Organisation, Specialisation, and Desires in the Big Men's Movement: Preliminary Research in the Study of Subculture-Formation," *Journal of Gay, Lesbian, and Bisexual Identity* 4, no. 3 (1999): 217-39.
59 Whitesel, *Fat Gay Men: Girth, Mirth, and the Politics of Stigma.*
60 Lawrence D. Mass, "Bears and Health" in *The Bear Book II: Further Readings in the History and Evolution of a Gay Male Subculture*, edited by Les K. Wright, 15-37 (New York: Haworth Press, 2001); Laurence Brown, "Fat Is a Bearish Issue" in *The Bear Book II: Further Readings in the History and Evolution of a Gay Male Subculture*, edited by Les K. Wright, 39-54 (New York: Haworth Press, 2001).
61 Nathaniel C. Pyle and Michael I. Loewy, "Double Stigma: Fat Men and Their Male Admirers" in *The Fat Studies Reader*, edited by Esther Rothblum and Sondra Solovay, 143-50 (New York: New York University Press, 2009).
62 Brendan Gough and Gareth Flanders, "Celebrating 'Obese' Bodies: Gay 'Bears' Talk About Weight, Body Image and Health," *International Journal of Men's Health* 8, no. 3 (2009): 235-53.
63 Chris Vargas and Greg Youmans, *Falling in Love...with Chris and Greg: Episode 3 - Food!* Oakland, CA, 2010. Digital Video.

encounters with individual men associated with Bear culture who are engaged with fat feminism. The opening up of NOLOSE to people of all genders also offers opportunities for developing fat lesbian and queer feminist hybrids with Bears. Femme-identified transmasculine fat feminism is also emerging through performance, in academia and though conversations.[64]

TRAVEL AND POWER

Travel cannot be taken at face value, it is also about power. Crossing national borders, for example from the US to the UK, as I have shown my genealogy of fat feminism to do, is not a neutral act. The US is a superpower whose massive influence is evident even at a small community level through recent feminist exports such as Riot Grrrl and LadyFest, both sites of transmission for fat activism. Britain's political and cultural subordination to the US imbues travelling fat feminist activism with power which is frequently taken for granted or constituted as benign. This is not to deny Britain's role as a coloniser, or European colonisation in the rest of the world. I am talking about cultural imperialism using the US as one example. Imperialism refers to unequal power relationships between cultures that reproduce the domination and subordination of one at the expense of another, and is produced through ideology, policy and cultural attitudes.[65]

This rendering of US power and influence is personal, it has helped

64 Wyatt Riot, "Wyatt Riot," http://www.originalplumbing.com/index.php/team/itemlist/user/507-wyattriot; James Burford and Sam Orchard, "Chubby Boys with Strap-Ons: Queering Fat Transmasculine Embodiment" in Queering Fat Embodiment, edited by Cat Pausé et al, 61-74 (Farnham: Ashgate, 2014); Glenn Marla, "Mister Marla," http://mistermarla.com/; Raju Rage and Mîran N, "Time Travelling Brown Bears: Intergenerational Interviews with Two Transmasculine Femmes of Color on Healing Justice," https://heimatkunde.boell.de/2013/05/01/time-travelling-brown-bears-intergenerational-interviews-two-transmasculine-femmes-color.
65 John Tomlinson, Cultural Imperialism: A Critical Introduction (London: Continuum, 1991); Lisa Duggan, The Twilight of Equality: Neoliberalism, Cultural Politics and the Attack on Democracy (Boston: Beacon Press, 2003).

to form me. I grew up in a working class British family who wanted
something similar to the post-war American Dream. As bright and
ambitious young people, my parents wanted meritocratic opportunities to
live the good lives that had always been denied them and their ancestors.
As an adult my views changed as I became more aware of systematic
abuse of human rights worldwide by the US and that country's relentless
self-aggrandisement. As this progressed I experienced a growing unease
thinking about how my fat activism is influenced by US imperialism.
I have written elsewhere about my ambivalence with being positioned
as "British" or as a foreigner performing Britishness by people in the
US because my relationship to the country where I was born is also an
uncomfortable one.[66] Recently I have wondered what might happen if
I am critical of the US. Can my fat activism still exist and flourish? At
the moment I don't know. Until other autonomous narratives appear
it will remain impossible to talk about fat activism without also being
subjected to US power.

When fat feminism and fat activism travel across international borders
that implicate the US, it is common for the fat activists "elsewhere" to be
diminished by the soft power of US cultural imperialism, Julia described
one such incident:

> One of the first discussions I had here [in Germany] about fat
> activist stuff was someone who'd recently arrived from the States,
> "I can't believe," sorry to do the accent but, whining, "there's no
> fat activism in the UK, what's wrong with people, I can't believe it,
> I'm astounded." I'm like, "That's not true actually," and I gave it to
> them. "So what's that going to achieve?" Totally snooty about it.
> I was like, "Look, it's not going to look the same, it's a completely
> different culture and, for the record, I'm not trying to emulate you
> either, why are you expecting it to look and function the same
> way? Of course it's not going to look and function the same way."
> Oh I phrased it very politely, however. (Julia)

66 Cooper, "A Queer and Trans Fat Activist Timeline."

Despite its travels to the UK and Australasia; or the existence of long-standing fat activist groups in non-Anglophone countries, such as Dicke in Germany, Allegro Fortissimo in France, Fat Positivity Belgium, or the defunct Vet Vrieg in The Netherlands; or work by Fat Studies scholars and activists based outside the US; or the possibility that critical work on fat exists elsewhere; the US is still presumed to be the centre of fat feminism and fat activism by those within and beyond that country.[67] US dominance is reproduced rather than challenged or resisted by activists and scholars. For example, Stephanie von Liebenstein argues that fat activism in Germany is different to that in other national contexts because of the legacy of post-war mass health initiatives following the Third Reich, yet her paper is orientated primarily towards the US, other German and European fat activists are overlooked, as though they do not exist, even though the journal that published her paper has an international editorial board of Fat Studies scholars and activists.[68] The study participants from outside the US reported to me that fat people elsewhere are constructed as happy recipients of US wisdom, they are not expected to speak back to cultural imperialism, achieve recognition in the US, or generate radical fat activism of their own, especially if they have not made themselves palatable to US audiences.

> I think from our experiences of going to American-based conferences, I think when either you or I have tried to say: "Things are different in other places" that is largely unacknowledged, because discussions of other places has quite low status. (Billy)

67 Barbara Bruno Altman's *History of the Health At Every Size® Movement* is a good example of how interventions outside the US and Canada barely get a mention in an allegedly definitive history. Barbara Bruno Altman, "The Haes® Files: History of the Health at Every Size® Movement," Association for Size Diversity and Health, http://healthateverysizeblog.org/2013/04/30/the-haes-files-history-of-the-health-at-every-size-movement-part-i/. Although she is writing primarily about Health At Every Size, I mention her here because of her inclusion of fat activism.
68 von Liebenstein, "Confronting Weight Discrimination in Germany."

Physical and technological barriers to creating a global movement are becoming less intrusive but the movement remains focused on US parochialism. International networks of fat activists are very poor, even where there is shared language, and it is naïve to presume that the internet has become an international free flow of ideas. Encounters with the US and the West are often violent in that people are coerced into adopting models that do not fit. There is evidence that fat activism exists beyond the West, for example in South America and Asia.[69] But evidence of fat activism is often based on reports that are filtered for Western audiences and within such a context it is difficult to say how local people might formulate fat activism. Western anthropological texts concerning alternative readings of fat in Othered cultures are invoked to show that fat hatred is not inevitable.[70] But there is scarce consideration of colonialism and its relationship to anthropology in these renderings and it is not enough just to take them at face value as a different form of fat activism.[71]

Xenophobia flourishes in a context where innate cultural superiority is assumed. I have been subjected to intrusive and ignorant comments about my cultural background at fat feminist gatherings in the US, for example through mimicking my accent, stereotyping me or assuming that I am less politically sophisticated than a local person. Racism also

69 Anonymous, "China Daily: 'Fat and Cool' Dance Group Performs," SINA Corporation, http://www.chinadaily.com.cn/photo/2007-09/14/content_6108764.htm; Laura, "Gorda!" http://gordazine.tumblr.com/; Krudas Cubensi, "Krudas Cubensi," http://www.krudascubensi.com/. See also the "Marshmallow Girl trend" from Japan as reported in the West.

70 Moral, "Letter: Fat Save Species," *Off Our Backs* 10, no. 3 (1980): 31; Don Kulick and Anne Meneley, *Fat: The Anthropology of an Obsession* (London: Penguin, 2005). Virgie Tovar writes a compelling account of her journey to The Cook Islands and its importance to her in becoming a fat activist, for example. Virgie Tovar, "Pecan Pie, Sex, and Other Revolutionary Things" in *Hot & Heavy: Fierce Fat Girls on Life, Love & Fashion*, edited by Virgie Tovar, 167-76 (Berkeley, CA: Seal Press, 2012).

71 See, for example differing accounts of indigenous fattening houses in Kulick Otobong et al, "Fattened by Force," *Trouble & Strife* no. 23 (1992): 8-9; Kulick and Meneley, *Fat: The Anthopology of an Obsession*; Shaw, *The Embodiment of Disobedience: Fat Black Women's Unruly Political Bodies*.

operates along these lines. For example, on Hiroshima Day in 2008[72] US
fat activist Marilyn Wann launched a project entitled *1000 Fat Cranes*.[73]
Having read a *New York Times* article about a Japanese policy to monitor
and fine employees based on their waist size, she embarked upon a
scheme to "send 1,000 Fat Cranes flying on a peace mission to Japan".[74]
This was an allusion to the powerful mythology of Sadako Sasaki, a girl
who died as a result of the Hiroshima atom bomb, and who sought to
fold 1000 paper cranes. This story has become a central narrative and
symbol of Japan's peace movement and is the basis of the Children's
Peace Monument in Hiroshima's Peace Memorial Park. Wann, who
had no contact with fat activists in Japan, proposed an adaptation of
this symbol, with an added fold to make the paper crane appear fat,
to encourage Japanese people to make peace with their bodies. The
project was launched with publicity and videos demonstrating the special
origami fold were circulated online.[75]

1000 Fat Cranes was an insensitive appropriation by people within
the US of a sacred symbol, which was then used to berate an anonymous
Other under the guise of "peace," launched on a day mourning the
catastrophic US military aggression in Japan. Critiques of the project
were slow to appear. Conversations took place first in private and then
in online public fora. One anonymous public criticism was offered,
presumably the author feared the social repercussions of writing under
their own name to point out that fat activists had a problem with racism.[76]

---

72 6 August.

73 Marilyn Wann, "1000 Fat Cranes," http://www.myspace.com/1000fatcranes.

74 Onishi Norimitsu, "Japan, Seeking Trim Waists, Measures Millions," *New York Times*, http://www.nytimes.com/2008/06/13/world/asia/13fat.html?_r=1&scp=1&sq=japanese%20government%20measure%20waist&st=cse&oref=slogin., Wann, "1000 Fat Cranes".

75 Lauren Gard, "Fat-Is-Beautiful Activist Marilyn Wann Protests Japan's Thinness Law," *SF Weekly*, http://www.sfweekly.com/2008-08-27/news/fat-is-beautiful-activist-marilyn-wann-protests-japan-s-thinness-law/; Marilyn Wann, "Fat Crane Video #1," http://www.myspace.com/video/1-000-fat-cranes/fat-crane-video-035-6/40192991#!/video/1000fatcranes/fat-crane-video-035-1/40184296.

76 Anonymous, "Rethinking 1000 Fat Cranes," http://blog.twowholecakes.com/2008/09/rethinking-1000-fat-cranes/.

1000 Fat Cranes was quietly abandoned soon after, and four years later Wann offered a public apology for it on her Facebook as part of another row about racism in fat activism.[77]

Fat feminism is grounded in anti-imperialism, its original proponents were part of the American civil rights movement and worked within a social model of mental health that sought to identify and challenge oppressive conditions within dominant culture. Early fat feminists affirmed the uses of racial and ethnic traditions, identity and experience as a fundament of fat liberation.[78] The radical feminism that initially enabled fat feminism to travel was similarly concerned with liberation struggles, and the question of how to live freely continues. In this way, fat feminism and fat activism can be regarded as de-colonising strategies because they are concerned with contesting the powerful and harmful learned, imposed occupation of fat oppression and obesity discourse on people.

But aspects of fat feminism, and other fat activist discourses, have the capacity to re-colonise people. Fat activists cannot be assumed to be anti-oppressive in other spheres, as Kris noted:

> Yeah, and even fat activists, like we're talking about, even though I would say that their goal is rarely, if ever, hopefully to reinforce the status quo, they probably aren't in terms of making fat bodies public, but they probably often are in terms of the status quo around race and class and things like that, right? So they may be making the fat body public but it may be coming through a very white, homogenous, heteronormative, hegemonic – whatever h-word you want to use – for a vision of reinforcing the status quo. (Kris)

77 Tara Shuai, "A Different Kind of Fat Rant: People of Color and the Fat Acceptance Movement," http://web.archive.org/web/20080919002110/http://www.fatshionista.com/cms/index.php?option=com_content&task=view&id=180&Itemid=9; Tara Shuai et al, "A Response to White Fat Activism from People of Color in the Fat Justice Movement," NOLOSE, http://www.nolose.org/activism/POC.php; Marilyn Wann, "I Appreciated Very Much This Post Today from Marianne Kirby on the Rotund and Also Comments There from Julia Starkey, Margarita Femme-Inista, and Others," Facebook, https://www.facebook.com/marilynwann.
78 Stein and Hoffstein, *Proceedings of the First Feminist Fat Activists' Working Meeting.*

Cultural imperialism and racism, for example, repeat patterns of colonisation and are a reminder that de-colonising fat bodies cannot be separated from the anti-colonial struggles by people of colour from which the metaphor springs. Fat activists are not only fighting for recognition in wider culture, they are fighting for recognition amongst each other.

One remedy for this could be that fat activists acknowledge the power of location and open themselves to other possibilities, as proposed by Impi:

> Ideally Americans, American fat scholars or American fat activists, would realise that because they are working in the United States it's always global, it's never local. Even though they want to believe that it's local it never is, and that's the reason they should always, when they're using their voice, they should always at least remember that they are using a global voice, they are not just using it for "our little group in Kansas" or whatever the typical place has to be, and whenever they're making big statements about fat and fatness and fat people, it would be also perhaps useful to remember that they are especially using a global voice.[...] They are fairly sensitive in that they always have this add, add whatever list, whether it's race, ethnicity, religion, class, blah blah blah, all this list, but then they fail to see that, ok, fatness is not just American fatness, or an American fat issue. (Impi)

But acknowledging the global implications of universalising US or Western identity is still no guarantee that fat activism and fat feminism will be able to become more fully anti-racist, anti-imperialist and anti-colonialist because there is little motivation for scholars and activists in the US to do so. Billy was less optimistic about change or accountability and suggested that fat activism in the US will continue to be upheld as the universal model, perhaps coercively:

> I can imagine a future where America becomes even more insular as new kinds of fat activisms around the world spring up, but, kind of, protecting the brand, could happen. (Billy)

Travelling fat activism has the capacity to expand intersectional ideas about what fat activism can be but problems arising through those travels also have the capacity to diminish it as it continues through its transnational journeys.

MOVEMENT AND STAGNATION

Because of its ability to travel, fat feminism has great potential in creating plural, hybrid spaces in discourses relating to fat. The discussions about gender at NOLOSE suggest that bridges can be built between ideologies. Unfortunately, fat feminism and, by extension, fat activism, has struggled to generate multiple narratives, despite travelling far and moving onto the internet. Fat activism with genealogical connections to fat feminism in London, Melbourne, Berlin or online today looks similar to that produced in Los Angeles in 1973. It is telling, for example, that *Fat Power* and *The Fat Liberation Manifesto*, both produced decades ago, maintain a contemporary feel; this is not evidence of unity, or merely a testimony to the strength of the writing, it also represents a discourse that has stagnated.[79] Fat activism is often as calcified as its proxies.

This exchange between Verity and I illustrates some of the frustrations of encountering concepts that have become tired clichés to us as experienced fat activists, and our hunger for more complexity within the movement.

> Charlotte: One of the things that I've been talking about fat activism with people, it seems like it's, the movement is like in a perpetual 101 state, people are so disconnected from the history and other people as well, generally, that it's always this, it is always this "love your body" kind of thing. If you've been involved in these ideas for any amount of time, it just bores you to tears, you're just not into it at all, and I think, I don't know, I think there are some

---

79 Louderback, *Fat Power*; Freespirit and Aldebaran, *Fat Liberation Manifesto*.

of us that would just, I mean where do we go from there? Where
do we go? What can the activism be?

The reason that it's been hard to move past the 101 stage, at least
it seems like that to me, I associate with a couple of things: one is
this idea that was certainly how I was introduced to fat politics,
"fat is healthy" right? So then, I mean and there was never-, also
with "love your body" it's such a static idea. So then, as we age, as
illness and death veers its ugly head as it is wont to do in the human
condition, and, then people got silent, they dropped off, you know,
I don't know, I mean some people might have thought they were
wrong, some people, it happened in all sorts of different ways but
it did not work with the received rhetoric. And "love your body"
like, one of the things that I have such a problem with that is, like,
your body changes every fucking second, so you can't, you can
love this body and then it'll be over in five minutes! There's got to
be something else that's more of a process or it's just impossible.
So, how is it? Has that changed? Really it's changed because we're
having this conversation. (Verity)

Verity speaks to the limitations of a popular fat activism that cannot
adequately encompass on-going pain, illness or frailty within its rhetoric,
or bodies in states of perpetual change. In the same vein, oppression
remains the theoretical starting point for fat feminist activism, but this
is not transformed into activism that is necessarily anti-oppression,
and neither does it fully account for fat activism that emerges through
pleasure, fun, or even privilege. Fat activism beyond white Western
Anglophone cultures remains unrecognised within the dominant parts
of the movement. Mayer's observation that fat feminism is a discourse
of isolation remains true: powerful kinship networks cannot always
be assumed, fat activists work under tremendous social pressure and
opprobrium, they are not always mutually supportive, and the discourse

remains usurped by its proxies elsewhere.[80] Instead of flourishing as expansive ways of knowing that people might scavenge and adapt for themselves, fat feminism and fat activism are more likely to be locked into reductive patterns of subordination based on controlled narratives. I will describe some of these tensions in the next chapter.

80 Mayer, "Foreword."

ACCESSING

Access refers to the ability of people to enter a place, somewhere they want to go. Access is important in fat activism because it is common for fat people to experience political, psychological, social and physical exclusion in the world. The ability to enter a place creates the potential to transform it. Fat activism is both dynamic and also suffers from a staleness. It is losing touch with its earlier radical energy and this is causing it to become inaccessible, especially to people who are already socially marginalised.

In this chapter I explore how some people and ideas have become more privileged and able to gain access to a public sphere than others in the movement. I start with a discussion about boundary-keeping when access is restricted to an idea of sameness, shared interests and safety. I describe how this affects individuals and how it contributes to the mood of the movement. I then develop this idea to talk about who gets pushed aside when neoliberal fat activism emphasises access rather than social transformation. This book is being published at a time when some fat activism is enjoying unprecedented visibility, but other kinds of fat activism and other fat activists are being pushed further out. These others are people who are already socially marginalised. A battle for fair representation and ownership is underway and those at the margins are rightly demanding space at the centre of the movement. I conclude with some comments about assimilation and argue that the distinctions between what is conservative and what is progressive in fat activism are not clear cut.

BEING THE SAME

Essentialism is the belief that all people sharing a trait will have things
in common that bind them; the trait indicates a particular sameness
and has political implications.[1] Boundary-making around sameness in
fat activism has been historically associated with creating an illusion of
safety, the creation of an actual place where people of shared identity
can gather without harassment from outsiders. Greta Rensenbrink's
account of body policing at the swimming pool exemplifies the historic
concerns with boundary-making and sameness.[2] Fat people typically
experience unwanted attention at the pool, but she describes a fat swim
where access was granted only to people weighing 200lbs (91kg or around
14st) or more in order to create an environment without harassment.
There were self-appointed monitors to enforce the rule and some thin
people were ejected. The value underpinning these actions was that to
be a fat activist, a safe person, one had to be a certain size.

When a line is drawn its boundaries become policed. Martha was
someone active in that milieu and would have been familiar with such
boundary enforcement. She expressed regrets about how it was invoked
to police fat activist membership elsewhere:

> I have to say, when I look back at it now from so many years later,
> we were arrogant and snotty, we were, although not everybody
> identified as a lesbian separatist, we really were in a certain way,
> lesbians, and you know like, "Ooh, straight women," and also
> we were pretty obnoxious about who was fat or who wasn't, and
> what came from that that was good was the kind of aesthetic
> commitment to fat bodies and seeing the beauty of fat women.
> But there wasn't, I heard later from a lot of women, that they felt
> like if they weren't 100% on board, they were going to get thrown

1 Richard L. Cartwright, "Some Remarks on Essentialism," *The Journal of Philosophy*
65 no. 20 (1968): 615-26.
2 Rensenbrink, "Fat's No Four-Letter Word."

off the boat, sort of. That's the obnoxious part. [...] There was no room for doubt. The little bit I understand about social movements, that's sort of typical. In the early days there's no room for doubt: you're with us or you're not. But of course life's a lot more grey than that, so that's what I think about that. (Martha)

Anna is someone who was "thrown off the boat". She described an incident that took place some years ago:

I heard of the, I think it was called the [fat feminist organisation] and I thought, "Ok, I'm starting to do academic-" this is early in my PhD career, "I'm starting to do actual writing about this stuff, let me see if I can present a paper." And I called and spoke to a woman who, thankfully I've completely forgotten who this person was, I've erased her identity so I can't, I'm not going to name names but it's like I can't remember the name. [My friend] knows who it is but won't tell me! And explained in my eager, fresh-faced, grad student way that I really wanted to do, you know, I was working on, god only knows what it was at the time but "I'd love to be part of this," and the woman asked me:, "Well, how much do you weigh?" and at that point, you know my weight goes up and down, at that point it was down, and so I said, "Oh, about 150 pounds [68kg, 10st] or so," and she said, you could hear the wall go up in her voice and she said, "We, we need to reserve space, you know, this is a safe space, we need to reserve space for people of size to present," and I said, "Ok," and then hung up and felt sad, and felt kind of pushed out by the place I had come from, the place I was certainly going back to, as I know my own physical trajectory. But, you know, also a little bit saddened by the whole, you know, very identity politics-y thing going on there. (Anna)

Whilst the impetus to create safe space is laudable, the reality of its policing is troubling. The distinction between insiders and outsiders is not necessarily clear. The perceived transgressors may be part of the very fabric of fat activism, they cannot be turned out or avoided, nor should they be. As Paz pointed out:

> What does it mean for folks who have lived a fat life, who have gone through weight loss surgery, and are connected to community? I feel like it's a similar question around gender stuff. You know, somebody who is in, say, a lesbian community, and has transitioned and identifies as a man, and that person also identifies as a lesbian, is a dyke, they're part of that community, maybe leadership in that community, they're already there. (Paz)

Safe space is not safe for everyone who might have a claim to it. People experience painful exclusion when they disrupt the tacit agreement of sameness, or are the wrong kind of people, or simply reflect intolerable taboos.

These exclusions affect individuals and also the movement as a whole. For example, early fat feminism developed a powerful critique of dieting and weight loss. The legacy of this critique is present today through some fat activists' attitudes towards weight loss surgery, for example.[3] More recent fat activists have promoted practises of "no diet talk," and "no fat talk," that is, a censure on language in order to maintain a culture in which it is safe to be fat.[4] This has been championed by various young women's associations and university sororities in the US, organisations that are politically mainstream.[5] The efficacy, dangers, ethics, political rationale for and health implications of dieting, weight

---

3 Karen Throsby, "'I'd Kill Anyone Who Tried to Take My Band Away': Obesity Surgery, Critical Fat Politics and the 'Problem' of Patient Demand," *Somatechnics* 2, no. 1 (2012): 107-26; NAAFA, "Naafa's Official Position: Weight-Loss Surgery," http://www.naafaonline.com/dev2/about/doc-weightLossSurgery.html.

4 The emphasis on policing language can be seen elsewhere in contemporary identity politics.

5 Bonnie Rochman, "Do I Look Fat? Don't Ask. A Campaign to Ban 'Fat Talk,'" *Time*, http://www.time.com/time/nation/article/0,8599,2025345,00.html; Natalie Perkins, "No Diet Talk; a Badge for Your Blog," http://www.definatalie.com/2011/11/18/no-diet-talk-a-badge-for-your-blog/.

loss drugs and surgery are not the issues at stake here, but rather what
happens to fat activism when they are positioned as a universal rallying
point and when weight loss becomes unspeakable.

Those who do not observe the taboo report instances of shunning and
shaming. Kerry had a gastric band and experienced rejection relating
to it within fat activism. She explained:

> What I've realised through my own experience, is that there's a
> hyper-morality and surveillance that operates in the fat acceptance
> and activist community in some quarters, that basically is
> seeking to reproduce, kind of, moral correctitude and propriety
> in its members and to, kind of, you know, to position them as
> morally and politically suspect, when they transgress any of the
> unwritten rules. (Kerry)

But you do not have to have had surgery to be under suspicion. Benjamin
recounted an incident which illustrates how a clear stance against weight
loss surgery by fat activists produces a culture of rumour-mongering
and paranoia.

> I had a really horrible experience with, I friend-requested [a fat
> activist] on Facebook. And she heard a rumour that I had weight
> loss surgery and I did not have weight loss surgery, and because
> she heard a rumour I had weight loss surgery she wouldn't accept
> my friend request. And I just wrote back and I was like, "I'm sorry
> that, based upon rumours, you won't accept my friend request,
> and that also makes me feel sad because I feel like the point of
> these social networking sites is that, you know, I think you do
> really badass work in the world and if I was friends with you I'd
> get to keep tabs on it. You know what, if you don't think that at
> over 300lbs, as a tranny dancer, I do enough in the world, you
> don't get to keep tabs on that too." I think it's just interesting. So
> I like to remind myself that I'm still a really big person. It's just
> interesting, I forget, I don't forget that I used to be larger, but

I have to, like, you know, I didn't do anything drastic. I was like, "Wow, that was really intense."

Charlotte: I'm so shocked by that.

Yeah, it was really hurtful because, but I mean, I also didn't have that response where I was like, "You know what? I didn't have weight loss surgery." But it was very awkward because I saw her and I was like, "I'm not, I can't be friendly to you." It was just like if someone heard a rumour I was gay or something. And what a weird rumour. It's so funny, actually I got my gall bladder removed, which was on the wrong side of your body as weight loss surgery, but now I get really nervous that that's what people think! I had laproscopic gall bladder removed, and I take my shirt off when I dance, and I think that people will think I've had weight loss surgery! Isn't that funny? (Benjamin)

Impi claimed that the perceived need for sameness and safety in fat activism reproduces cycles of exclusion.

I do understand the need to separate yourself from, like, "Ok, this is our thing and we identify as fat people and we are in this group." Well, ok, I think one part of it is to make the separation between us and all this, that, "we are the ones who are in with this knowledge and in with this crowd and you are not." Like paying back all the times when you are, you have felt, left outside. And sometimes I don't think that people realise what they are doing, that they are feeding the same cycle of just wanting to leave other people out of our revolution, because this is our thing. And, well, in any case I would be really careful about branding other, some people, as not part of this group, or others as belonging to it self-evidently because that's not the case. (Impi)

The surveillance and threat of exclusion that Kerry, Benjamin and Impi described contributes to a climate in which critical speech becomes risky, culminating in the possibility of retribution and excommunication. During the process of interviewing people for this study, for example, some people were hesitant to give critical comments when asked about the types of fat activism they disliked. This response is typical:

> Charlotte: I'm interested in the kinds of fat activism that really turn you off, that you think are just either a waste of time or that irritate you. What doesn't work?

> Yeah well, you know it's like I do hesitate to answer that because I um, I don't want to ever put, so I would ask that you, are you, you wouldn't attach my name to, you can say generally "some people said this," but I do not want you to say "[name] said this". (A participant who did not wish to be named, even via a pseudonym)

Adiva argued that these tensions are an understandable by-product of a situation where fat people are under attack.

> I think at the same time, the people in the trenches who are really getting the barbed end of the fat hatred on a daily basis, I mean like on a second-by-second basis, like, we're not going to be perfect people, and we're going to have times of nastiness and rage and unpleasantness, and we're going to write things that aren't perfect, and I think that's all part of just understanding that we are under immense pressure. (Adiva)

The social pressure under which fat activists act cannot be discounted, yet there is a tremendous cost when some positions and people are rendered more necessary than others. That this goes on in a liberation movement could be considered a queer paradox, or evidence that some people really are expendable; it could also be argued that these sacrifices are inexcusable.

GENTRIFYING FAT

In drawing out some historical fat feminisms in this book I have shown that fat activism reflects the times in which it is produced. It is easier to see this when looking at the past but it is also happening in the present. I have argued that my genealogy of fat activism comes from the civil rights movement, radical feminism as well as socialism and other radical politics. Today, fat activism is more likely to be framed by neoliberalism because now is a time in which this ideology is ascendant, even within the alternative cultures that spawned fat activism.[6] This is another way in which it has travelled.

Neoliberalism is an economic philosophy rooted in capitalism that is predominant in the West and is being exported to the rest of the world as part of globalisation. Confusingly, neoliberalism has meant different things at different times but I use it here to mean an emphasis on individualism rather than collectivity; a survival of the fittest mentality; a belief in every man(sic) for himself; the end of public resources owned by everybody for the sake of private resources owned by a few. These values can be seen in strategies such as demolishing welfare and reducing the role of government, deregulating business, Austerity and privatisation. Neoliberal describes much of what is going on in the West today, including political shifts to the right, the polarising of rich and poor, and the emphasis on profit. Lisa Duggan argues that neoliberalism shifts resources away from marginalised people at the bottom of the heap. For her this has happened through the development of more conservative agendas in LGBT identity politics, for example regarding inclusion in and acceptance of the institutions of marriage

---

6 Neoliberalism is also a defining feature of obesity discourse. Julie Guthman and Melanie DuPuis, "Embodying Neoliberalism: Economy, Culture, and the Politics of Fat," *Environment and Planning D: Society and Space* 24 (2006): 427-48; Guthman, "Teaching the Politics of Obesity: Insights into Neoliberal Embodiment and Contemporary Biopolitics"; Helene A. Shugart, "Consuming Citizen: Neoliberating the Obese Body," *Communication, Culture & Critique* 3 (2010): 105-26.

and the military instead of their abolition or reform.[7]

I want to use the concept of gentrification to develop my discussion of fat activism and access within neoliberalism. I think of gentrification as what happens when activists gain access to power *but fail or decline to transform it*. Gentrification refers to the manner by which wealthy incomers displace poorer communities through friendly coercion and the appearance of progress through social cleansing and raised property prices.[8] Incomers appropriate spaces as their own to the extent that older claims to the space are erased or distorted and sold back to the community. I am using gentrification here not as a geographer's term to describe a city's development but as a metaphor. I am following Sarah Schulman's use of gentrification in her discussion of the erasure of queer and trans people with AIDS in New York City.[9] In her definition I substitute "social movement" for neighbourhood and city:

> To me, the literal experience of gentrification is a concrete replacement process. Physically it is an urban phenomena: the removal of communities of diverse classes, ethnicities, races, sexualities, languages, and points of view from the central neighbourhoods of cities, and their replacement by more homogenised groups. With this comes the destruction of culture and relationship, and this destruction has profound consequences for the future lives of cities.

7 Duggan, *The Twilight of Equality*. That some fat people are allowed access and some are denied is reminiscent of Gayle Rubin's "Charmed Circle" which illustrates, in terms of sexuality, those who are socially acceptable and those who are not. Rubin, "Thinking Sex: Notes for a Radical Theory of the Politics of Sexuality."

8 Christina B. Hanhardt shows how an idea of politically strategic sameness is connected to gentrification through the push to create safe urban spaces for rich white LGBT people. Christina B. Hanhardt, *The Safe Space: Gay Neighborhood History and the Politics of Violence* (Durham, NC: Duke University Press, 2013).

9 Sarah Schulman, *The Gentrification of the Mind: Witness to a Lost Imagination* (Oakland, CA: University of California Press, 2012).

I have talked about people being denied access to fat activism because of their size, either by being too thin or having lost weight through surgery. But, as Schulman points out, exclusion and erasure brought about by neoliberalism and gentrification are tactics that further marginalise people along the lines of gender, class, race and disability and many other factors and intersections.[10] Thus Sara Auerbach and Rebekah Bradley propose that the fat dyke is a heroic figure within a queer space but within an assimilationist and gentrified LGBT culture identified with dominant cultural values she becomes just another woman with a weight problem.[11] Amber Hollibaugh notes that gentrifiers refuse to see those whom they displace.[12] In the process of gaining access to the mainstream, some people, the marginal people, tend to be sacrificed.[13] In this context I think of gentrification as a vector for loss, erasure and politically convenient forgetting that is happening in some of the most visible forms of fat activism concerned with consumerism, professionalisation, supremacy and healthism.

10   Homonationalism is another useful term concerning neoliberalism to consider here; popularised in academia by Jasbir Puar, it refers to the process by which minority sexual groups identify with dominant cultural groups at the expense of the more marginal members of those minority groups. Jasbir K. Puar, *Terrorist Assemblages: Homonationlism in Queer Times* (Durham, NC: Duke University Press, 2007).

11 Sara Auerbach and Rebekah Bradley, "Resistance and Reinscription: Sexual Identity and Body Image among Lesbian and Bisexual Women" in *Looking Queer: Body Image and Identity in Lesbian, Bisexual, Gay, and Transgender Communities*, edited by Dawn Atkins, 27-36 (Philadelphia, PA: Haworth Press, 1998).

12 Amber Hollibaugh, "Queers without Money: They Are Everywhere. But We Refuse to See Them," http://www.villagevoice.com/2001-06-19/news/queers-without-money/.

13 A recent special issue of *Fat Studies: An Interdisciplinary Journal of Body Weight and Society* reveals how entrenched this problem is, even when intersectionality is the focus: "The contributions in this issue [on intersectionality] fail to address many important intersections. All of the authors, for example, hail from Western cultures (United States, the United Kingdom, and New Zealand). And issues such as race, class, and ability, are largely neglected in this offering." Cat Pausé, "X-Static Process: Intersectionality within the Field of Fat Studies," *Fat Studies: An Interdisciplinary Journal of Body Weight and Society* 3, no. 2 (2014): 80-85.

CONSUMERISM AND GENDER

Fatshion is central to fat activism today and closely tied to body positive rhetoric within the movement. Fashion can help people to be more accepting of their bodies. Businesses making clothes in larger sizes have had vested interests in selling an idealised version of fat embodiment for many years, and this began to be contextualised as activism through small fashion businesses owned and run by fat activists from the 1980s onwards. Lauren Downing Peters suggests that fashion was derided by earlier fat activists because of a feminist aversion to it within a politics critical of beauty.[14] I disagree with this because of evidence from my *Timeline* project and in *Shadow on a Tightrope*; fat feminists were interested in fashion from the beginning.[15] But it wasn't until 2004 when Amanda Piasecki coined the term *Fatshionista* for an online community that the activist implications of fat and fashion could be expressed on a mass scale that was also connected to the growth of social media.

As someone who had worked in corporate plus size retail, Piasecki wanted to develop a community discussion about fat, fashion and politics that paid attention to working class people, queers and people of colour. *Fatshionista* was initially a product of queer femme community, where adornment was a means of survival and visibility, and where people came from traditions of using whatever resources were available to them. *Fatshionista* established femme identity as central to the movement, and developed a powerful collective counter-aesthetic to mainstream renderings of fat abjection.[16]

What began as a small-scale discussion amongst friends soon grew into a hugely popular online community to the extent that its name

14 Lauren Downing Peters, "Queering the Hourglass: Beauty and New Wave Fat Activism" in *Beauty: Exploring Critical Issues* (Oxford, UK, 2013).

15 Cynthia Riggs, "Fat Women and Clothing: An Interview with Judy Freespirit" in *Shadow on a Tightrope: Writings by Women on Fat Oppression*, edited by Lisa Schoenfielder and Barb Wieser, 139-43 (Iowa City: Aunt Lute, 1983).

16 Afful and Ricciardelli, "Shaping the Online Fat Acceptance Movement: Talking About Body Image and Beauty Standards"; Downing Peters, "Queering the Hourglass: Beauty and New Wave Fat Activism."

became a generic term for any iteration of fat and fashion. The group's popularity exposed problems within the concept. Anna named these as unquestioned ideologies of consumerism and citizenship within fat activism and fashion.

> There's a kind of consumer-citizenship, I guess, that is centred around fashion, like a post-feminist consumer-citizenship centred around fashion that, you know, I'm intrigued by, but I think has a fairly assimilatory tendency to it. (Anna)

Hannah talked about her experience in how this consumer-citizenship manifested itself as a means of speaking back to corporations, and how it ended up being appropriated.

> So in American culture at least, a lot of the ways that middle class girls intersect with or have a rite of passage is by the body project, it's all about figuring out how you relate your body to the world and what that means, and often that means obsessing about clothes and how you present yourself, and middle class fat women are really denied this experience in a lot of ways. What I found with [a fatshion community I was involved with] is that, as time went on, it became this substitute for a body project for women who had never had those experiences. And so it was a rift between people who actually wanted to talk about the body and what it meant, and people who wanted to get validated for their outfits. [...] And eventually I got really embarrassed by it [...]. I was like, "This is not about my values at all," this was about American consumerism and mostly white women being denied the opportunity to have consumerism in the way that they wanted. And it's a free market research tool for all these companies [...]. I felt horrified by it. (Hannah)

This account reflects the capitalist strategy of treating countercultural expression as a resource to take over and market back to consumers as a marker of identity. Images that represent a counter-aesthetic are not immune to this appropriation, they enable corporations to maintain their grip on the market by appearing to be relatable or well-informed.[17] *Fatshionista* became a marketing tool not only in its original form as a LiveJournal community but also through the activism it sparked. Fatshion bloggers proliferated, the more popular of whom were snapped up by corporations looking to create "brand ambassadors" to re-sell fatshion back to their customers.[18] Whilst fatshion as activism became part of an imperative to create profit, what was lost in this process was the original call to critique fatshion put forward by queer femmes, many of whom were working class as well as being people of colour.

In their paper exploring feminist consumerism and fat activism, Josée Johnston and Judith Taylor describe how grassroots activists have traditionally been understood as critics of consumerism and corporate appropriation.[19] Indeed, community clothing swaps, The Flea and the Big Bum Jumble continue to provide a space that is critical of corporate commodification. These are very small moments compared to the consumerism of fatshion. But a study by Daiane Scaraboto and Severino Joaquim Nunes Pereira argues that corporate commodification *is* activism.[20] Not only does fatshion and social media enable activists to develop positive self-identities, it also allows them to influence the market.[21] This proposal by Liz illustrated how capitalism has become an acceptable tool for activists, not only in fatshion but also in alternatives to weight loss.

17 Johnston and Taylor, "Feminist Consumerism and Fat Activists."

18 Kelly Faircloth, "Fatshion Police: How Plus-Size Blogging Left Its Radical Roots Behind," *The New York Observer*, http://betabeat.com/2013/02/fatshion-plus-size-bloggers-amanda-piasecki-marianne-kirby-gabrielle-gregg/.

19 Johnston and Taylor, "Feminist Consumerism and Fat Activists."

20 Daiane Scaraboto and Severino Joaquim Nunes Pereira, "Rhetorical Strategies of Consumer Activists: Reframing Market Offers to Promote Change," *Brazilian Administration review* 10, no. 4 (2013): 389-414.

21 Daiane Scaraboto and Eileen Fischer, "Frustrated Fatshionistas: An Institutional Theory Perspective on Consumer Quests for Greater Choice in Mainstream Markets," *Journal of Consumer Research* 39 no. 6 (2013): 1234-1257.

Fat hatred is fuelled by capitalism because these companies create products that are all about making fat people skinny, but it's really about making money, it's not about your health, obviously. But we don't have a comparable thing to hang our little hat on […] I think the answer is not not doing that [building fat activist businesses], because we can't not do it, like messages are driven by money, even if they're driven by beliefs […] And I think that things, I mean they have to actually have a positive effect on people's lives, but I think that, you know, if you were choosing like paying, whatever, 19.99 a month to be on Weight Watchers, and go through that experience of paying 19.99 a month to be in some kind of Health At Every Size experience that makes you feel good, you know it's going to have a direct impact. That person wants to spend 19.99 for relief of something. (Liz)

Using capitalism as a basis for activism illustrates how, within the gentrification of fat activism it is access rather than social transformation that has become the main motivator. This is also gendered: it is women and feminine-of-centre people who are producing these forms of activism as well as being fodder for appropriation. What started as resistance and critique by people with limited capital to participate in neoliberal culture is now a buying opportunity that further excludes those who are too poor to participate.

PROFESSIONALISATION AND CLASS

Professionalisation refers to the social process in which an activity previously undertaken without restriction becomes the domain of professionals. The purpose of this is to raise standards and be legible to large institutions, but it also has the effect of keeping people out. I understand this as a class issue because without the financial and cultural capital to access these professionalised resources, built on previously freely available community knowledge, admission becomes restricted. What is also being gentrified through professionalisation is a raucous and powerful fat activist voice that I associate with the impolite, the unrefined, the distasteful and the unclassy.

Professionalisation happens when people become organised in groups designed to protect the profession. These groups establish norms and standards. For example in 2010 the concept Health At Every Size was trademarked by Think Tank, a group of health professionals and activists that meets in San Leandro, California. This was done so that weight loss corporations could not appropriate HAES but the act also removed the concept from public ownership and self-appointed its controllers as moral guardians.[22] It is important that professionals are separate from amateurs and that being a professional confers more status than being an amateur. Professional bodies decide who can be part of the group and who is excluded, they are gatekeepers. Professionalised groups might also impose qualifications and certification. This can have the effect of killing off the amateur, even though the work of amateurs is what professionalisation has been built on. For example, Health At Every Size grew from activists talking and organising around their dismal experiences of health care and can be found in the earliest Fat Underground publications.[23] HAES has been adopted to some extent by some health practitioners and part of this process has been its professionalisation, which means that it is no longer a grassroots affair. Social justice is not always present in interpretations of HAES and fat activism is now a dwindling part of the philosophy it helped to bring about. Professionalisation is thus implicated in the production of hierarchies and elites. This means that knowledge can become closed off in institutions, made subject to fees or it may require special skills to find.

Social cleansing is central to gentrification and so it is too to the professionalisation of fat activism. This can be seen through the use of language. "Fat" is too abrasive and politicised in this context, so the more

22 Jacqui Gingras and Charlotte Cooper, "Down the Rabbit Hole: A Critique of the ® in Haes®," *Journal of Critical Dietetics* 1, no. 3 (2013): 2-5.
23 Aldebaran, *Health of Fat People: The Scare Story Your Doctor Won't Tell You* (Los Angeles/New Haven, CT: The Fat Underground/Largesse Fat Liberation Archives, 1974).

anodyne and less specific "weight" is substituted. Instead of fatphobia or fat hatred, which confer some of the emotional experience of being fat, "weight stigma" and "weight bias" become preferred terms. No fear, hatred, rage, oppression or other untidy emotion is allowed to clutter these fascinating and dispassionate debates.[24] The discussion is no longer about fat people's struggle for survival, our feelings are unsophisticated, inferior, perplexing and embarrassing. Fat Studies is appropriated and whitewashed into "Critical Weight Studies."[25] These terms gain currency because of the perceived professional power of those wielding them, a power that is often bound up in the users' normative embodiment and sense of entitlement to define the terms of being fat. Liat commented on this process:

> It's interesting, it's like in a way the movement's at their most radical, they kind of have to become palatable for the mainstream, and so I see all those people as sort of co-opting the lesbian feminism, the radical, most radical stuff, and really most of it is language, you know where fat liberation, lesbian fat liberationists talk about "fat and liberation," and then it becomes "size and body image" and they're saying kind of the same things but they're making it

24 Keep in mind that being fat is often associated with particular emotive states, shame being especially central. Erdman Farrell, *Fat Shame*; Jeannine A. Gailey, "Fat Shame to Fat Pride: Fat Women's Sexual and Dating Experiences," *Fat Studies: An Interdisciplinary Journal of Body Weight and Society* 1, no. 1 (2012): 114-27. Fat people also undertake considerable emotional labour in managing stigma in the workplace and beyond. Goffman, *Stigma*; Arlie Russel Hochschild, *The Managed Heart: Commercialisation of Human Feeling* (Berkeley and Los Angeles: University of California Press, 2003). This is the affective work of politeness in the face of hate, the work of ignoring and "rising above" as a survival tool.

25 In recent years a small number of academics have used Critical Obesity Studies and Critical Weight Studies interchangeably with Fat Studies, a term that emerged through fat activist community, for no clear reason. Deborah Lupton writes that critical is the operative term yet there is little critical engagement with how the terms uphold euphemisms for fat, erase the struggle for self-determination and knowledge ownership by fat people and maintain a disconcerting alliance with obesity discourse. Lupton, *Fat*. I would assume that the word fat is itself the critique and that the use of 'critical' is superfluous.

palatable for middle America, or whoever, and of course lesbians are discredited because we're a fringe element, and who would listen to us? (Liat)

Queer and lesbian feminist contributions to fat activism have been overlooked or actively erased through a professionalised gentrification. For example, Sue Dyson quotes extensively from the *Fat Dykes Statement*, but fails to mention its original title, excises references to lesbians, and does not attribute it to one of the lesbian workshops at the 1989 Fat Women's Conference in London where it was produced, even though a full credited version was published two years previously.[26]

Part of the way in which professionalisation becomes a class privileged domain is by the displacement of fat people by those who are normatively-sized. Barbra pointed out that normatively-sized fat activists are often constructed as "allies."

I suppose I'm thinking that allies is used as a, "Well, what are we going to do with the thin people? We'll call them allies" [...] and then we can accept them into the fold. (Barbra)

The construction of allies has enabled more people to participate in a movement that has struggled with boundary-keeping concerning size, as I pointed out earlier in this chapter. The concept of allies implies that there is a more authentic subject position within the movement, that of fat people. But this is problematic because it also suggests a process of boundary-making and policing. Later on I will discuss how I approach the issue of making mixed fat activist spaces without resorting to this concept. Allies are constructed as secondary beings, but they do not always know their place! The tension between having thin privilege and being de-centred is a complicated one to negotiate and privilege often trounces the situation. Fat people who are activists are complicit

26 Smith, "Creating a Politics of Appearance"; Sue Dyson, *A Weight Off Your Mind: How to Stop Worrying About Your Body Size* (London: Sheldon Press, 1991).

with this at times. Barbra also referred to an idea that normatively-sized people are in a better position to speak about fat than fat people because they are less likely to be devastated by a public attack on their beliefs.

> I think thin, having thin people involved, especially in that area is a bonus because it's the whole thing of like, "Well, they're not going to listen to us because we're the fatties and there's something wrong with us. But you don't have anything invested in that, you're not trying to explain that your body is ok, it's not a personal thing." (Barbra)

Abigail Saguy acknowledges this power:

> Because of my relative thinness, I am often unfairly considered a more objective, and thus more credible, commentator on debates over fatness than if I were fat, in that people assume I have no personal axe to grind.[27]

The problem here is that activists are relying on thinner people's privilege instead of transforming public spaces so that everybody can access them.

Anyone can be a fat activist regardless of their size. But this position is complicated because there are differences in experience, access, privilege and power that are built on the relationship between fatness and normativity.[28] These expressions of power and privilege need to be acknowledged when normatively-sized people pursue or assume prominent roles in the movement, whether or not they are positioned as allies. Creating professionalised spaces addressing fat where thinner

27 Saguy, *What's Wrong with Fat?*
28 Recent examples in my experience of these differences: a thin ally's study of fat people nets them a fancy job; a group of normatively-sized scholars receive major funding for their Fat Studies projects; a thin academic publishes an expensive book about fat activism; another invites a fat person into their work, unpaid, as a legitimising community-engagement token; fat people's contributions are considered less important or lay compared to those offered by thin people at a major conference, even though they are built on years of experience and scholarship.

people predominate is problematic. This exclusion is not usually premeditated, more a product of the assumption that fat people are not agents or narrators of our own lives, or capable of contributing usefully. It reflects the pervasive absence of fat people in obesity discourse. The displacement of fat people's voices occurs in settings that are already exclusive and professionalised, where access by lower class people is limited, for example the academy. Taking the absence of fat people for granted in professionalised spaces is not socially transformative. Neither is taking and transforming grassroots stories for professional gain, cleaning them up to make them more palatable to the powerful, or mystifying them through professionalised jargon and erasure.

SUPREMACY AND RACE

Black women are key figures in resisting fatphobic, sexist and racist normativity,[29] but the gentrification of fat activism entails the erasure of people of colour from the movement and their replacement with a logic of white supremacy. Because of white supremacy and racism, fat activists face many difficulties developing broader anti-oppressive standards in the movement, and emphasising the experiences of people of colour and other marginalised groups.[30]

This displacement permeates through politically convenient forgetting in the historicising of fat activism. People of colour and people from minority ethnic backgrounds have been part of fat activism since the beginning and the movement itself was initiated through a relationship with civil rights.[31] Judy Freespirit mentions that many of the early fat

29 Shaw, *The Embodiment of Disobedience: Fat Black Women's Unruly Political Bodies.*
30 Margaret K. Bass, "On Being a Fat Black Girl in a Fat-Hating Culture" in *Recovering the Black Female Body: Self-Representations by African American Women*, edited by Michael Bennett and Vanessa D. Dickerson, 219-30 (New Brunswick, NJ: Rutgers University Press, 2001); Shuai, "A Different Kind of Fat Rant."
31 Charlotte Cooper, "Charlotte Cooper and Judy Freespirit in Conversation, June 2010," http://obesitytimebomb.blogspot.com/2010/09/charlotte-cooper-and-judy-freespirit-in.html.

feminists were civil rights activists in the US, and fat activism owes a debt to that movement as well as contemporary global struggles for self-determination and anti-colonialism. However, the people of colour within the civil rights movement who created a context from which early fat activism could develop are invisible and undocumented, as far as I could find during the research for this book.

White supremacy and cultural erasure also operate through present day fat activism. This supremacy is present when white people become those most entitled to speak and when their experience is universalised. In 2012 an anti-child obesity poster campaign was launched in Georgia in the US featuring portraits of fat children accompanied by anti-obesity slogans. Andrea Shaw points out that fat black women are symbols of failure in white supremacist culture, thus racialised and working class people are invariably the face of the obesity epidemic and are vulnerable to interventions that arise as a result of that rhetoric.[32] The *I Stand* project, instigated by Marilyn Wann, created posters of fat activists with slogans offered in solidarity with the children depicted in the campaign. At least 389 of these posters were created and disseminated through social media. The original campaign targeted African American communities whilst the subjects in the hundreds of fat activist posters were overwhelmingly white Westerners. The fat activist posters were produced for the benefit of a community that was not included in the project which, ironically, reflects how anti-obesity policy is also usually produced. Scant attention was paid to the impact of the project on the African American children of Georgia and instead *I Stand* became a missive to an idea of a universalised child from a universalised white Western body of activists. Nuances of race and class were lost, the white Western voice was presumed to speak for all with authority. Initially those invested with the project were defensive when called to account for these discrepancies. But when a group of people of colour wrote an

32 Shaw, *The Embodiment of Disobedience: Fat Black Women's Unruly Political Bodies*; Shuai et al, "A Response to White Fat Activism from People of Color in the Fat Justice Movement".

open letter about the project Wann issued a public apology and closed it down.[33] Yet *I Stand* remains a source of pride for many fat activists, an example of the robust use of social media and an exciting example of community mobilisation.[34] An awkward silence preponderates when the spectre of racism is invoked. The anti-racist critique of *I Stand* was met with a ferocious denial of racism by fat activists online.[35]

White supremacy in fat activism also precludes the potential contributions of people of colour to the movement in the future by establishing white people as its only legitimate agents. An example of this happened at a workshop I attended in Berlin in 2012 for European fat activists. The main event, a planned part of the workshop, was a protest at Alexanderplatz, a large and historic public space for International No Diet Day. A table was set up laden with sweets and snacks and leaflets were handed out to passers-by. All of the workshop participants were white. There is a Roma community present at Alexanderplatz. Women and children in this space make a living through hustling and begging. Popular perception of them is very negative. Members of this community approached the table like all the other passers-by, presumably hoping to be given some of the treats that were being handed out and to find out what was going on. The workshop leader shooed them away and covered the food with her hands, saying, "This is not for you." This happened several times. She did not shoo away any other kinds of people. Kay Hyatt and I witnessed this, took food (including some that had ironically been coded as prized, special and restricted) and gave it to the Roma women and children who

33 "A Response to White Fat Activism from People of Color in the Fat Justice Movement"; Marilyn Wann, "Apology...", http://istandagainstweightbullying.tumblr.com/.

34 Anonymous, "Fat Kids United," https://fatkidsunited.wordpress.com/; Cat Pausé, "Causing a Commotion: Queering Fat in Cyberspace" in *Queering Fat Embodiment*, edited by Cat Pausé et al, 75-88 (Farnham: Ashgate, 2014).

35 Shannon Russell, "Shut Down," http://fiercefatties.com/2012/03/22/shut-down/. See Latoya Peterson on white refusal of intersectionality in fat activism. Latoya Peterson, "Intersectionality Extends to Fat Acceptance Too!" *Racialicious*, http://www.racialicious.com/2008/03/24/intersectionality-extends-to-fat-acceptance-too/.

wanted it. Kay confronted the workshop leader, saying that it was unacceptable to deny people and that she was being racist, but she refused to engage, racism had nothing to do with this protest or the workshop.[36] The workshop leader tried to compromise by saying that she would distribute any leftover food to the Roma people at the end of the event, but this turned out later not to be true. Kay and I left. One of the other workshop participants grumbled to us but took no action, the others said nothing. At a party for the event that evening, leftover food from the event was thrown around and left for rubbish.[37] Meanwhile, the protest drew considerable media coverage in Germany with pictures showing white people holding placards and extolling the benefits of Health At Every Size. This was the source of conversation the following day, not the treatment of the Roma people, and attempts to talk about what had happened were shut down. The group did not want to reflect or change.

It is not just the hand-covering, shooing away and denial that is shocking in this story, but the profound and automatic assumption of white supremacy underpinning the event and the gathering. Earlier on in the workshop there had been some moments (a "tribal" dance and a reference to cannibalism) which hinted that racism was acceptable. Even if the Roma women and children had been given sweets and information and included in the event it would not have altered the overriding attitude towards them, before they approached the table they had already been conceived of as subordinate to the white fat activist majority. This was understood in the workshop group as normal

36 Jenny Ellison's comments about fat activism, whiteness and a lack of an intersectional analysis resonate here: "While there is some evidence that they were aware of different cultural perspectives on fatness, questions about race were often met with confusion or discomfort. Many of my participants saw fat as the central unifying characteristic of their groups and had not considered that most members were also white." Ellison, "Weighing In: The 'Evidence of Experience' and Canadian Fat Women's Activism."

37 I return to Sara Ahmed's figure of the killjoy here. Ahmed, *The Promise of Happiness*. The cheerful consensus was coerced at the expense of queer, migrant, "extremist", awkward voices, it was built on suppression of difference and dissent, hence this jolly party was not at all "happy".

and acceptable. Without questioning this and making fundamental changes to the way that fat activism was configured, "inclusion" would have been another transmission of supremacy. But at the protest, ownership of public space was assumed by virtue of the workshop participant's whiteness and the presumed illegitimacy of the Roma in being there was understood because they were people of colour, even though on our journey to Alexanderplatz earlier in the day we had passed by monuments to Roma genocide during the Holocaust. They were simply regarded as unacceptable opportunistic beggars, not really human or people with a claim to the city. The group replaced a racially-mixed space with a white monoculture under the guise of fat activism. They pushed the Roma further out and insulted them. The group had the opportunity to transform what International No Diet Day or fat activism might look like in front of the media but they failed to do so because of an investment in white supremacy and a lack of an anti-oppressive imagination. They represented fat activism and replicated a self-fulfilling prophecy that the movement is white and that only these people get to become activists, to speak, to benefit from it. They assumed that Roma people would never have anything useful to contribute to a conversation about fat and that fat activism is rightfully controlled and dictated by white people.

HEALTHISM AND DISABILITY

Healthism refers to the idea that health is a moral project that is the responsibility of the individual.[38] Here, health is not merely the absence of illness, it is about presenting yourself to the world as glowingly well, athletic, able-bodied and full of vitality.

Neoliberalism functions through the actions of productive citizens

---

38 Petr Skrabanek, *The Death of Humane Medicine and the Rise of Coercive Healthism*, (Bury St Edmonds: The Social Affairs Unit, 1994); Nikolas Rose, *Powers of Freedom: Reframing Political Thought* (Cambridge: Cambridge University Press, 1999); Julianne Cheek, "Healthism: A New Conservatism?" *Qualitative Health Research* 18, no. 7 (2008): 974-82.

who never get ill and can work until they die without any state support. In a privatised society where universal access to free or cheap healthcare is not guaranteed, and where the state refuses to assume the burden of care, it is imperative that people take personal responsibility for their bodies, assuming at the very least an appearance of health.[39] Within the politics of Austerity, fat people are treated as a drain on scarce resources rather than resources becoming compromised through political programmes of funding cuts.[40] Where there is no safety net of welfare, people face great pressure to be fit for the marketplace, to present themselves as competitively employable, to be winners. Fat people represent failed citizens within this frame, the slow, unwell, undisciplined and unemployable losers in the race of life whose only chance of betterment is by participating within neoliberal health regimes.

Gentrified fat activism is healthist in that it elevates some kinds of bodies over others; instead of the belief that all bodies are valuable, only the good, compliant ones matter. This happens through activism that is concerned with showing that fat people are as healthy and therefore as morally good as normatively-sized people. Kathleen LeBesco refers to the "will to innocence" in fat activism, meaning the strategic denial that fat people are responsible for their fatness.[41] Here fat activists present themselves as correctly-behaved, blame-free, healthist citizens with regard to their exercise and eating habits. It is a gentrified fat activism of the exceptional individual rising above an assumed morass of the less or unworthy. This creates fat activism that quickly becomes intolerable and untenable for many people including those who are superfat, unfit, unhealthy, or chronically ill. It is not only intolerable but these groups cannot be tolerated. Not coincidentally, these are also people with the lowest socioeconomic status. Those who cannot uphold healthism in

39 David Harvey, *A Brief History of Neoliberalism* (Oxford: Oxford University Press, 2007).
40 Graham-Leigh, *A Diet of Austerity.*
41 LeBesco, *Revolting Bodies.*

fat activism tend to leave the movement. They are formulated as the problem, not healthism.

Zoë Meleo-Erwin argues that fat activists should develop critical approaches to normativity, especially within health.[42] This is likely to be a long time coming because of the depth of belief that to be fat is to be unhealthy and therefore morally suspect within neoliberalism.[43] Healthcare workers could be agents of change[44] but Eve described how their professional identities often surpass their associations with activism:

> One of the things that I think is really not said often enough is that Health At Every Size is a specific response to the specific vehicle of oppression of fat people around health. It is not a comprehensive fat activism analysis. It suffers from a kind of myopia, or a lot of the people who are sort of doing HAES are specifically responding to that stereotype of fat being unhealthy, and not really broadening out to a larger focus that's way beyond health in some of the analysis. And so I understand that the tensions exist there. They're focusing so much on health still, and we're doing that partly because we're healthcare professionals, a lot of us, who are really trying to mount some resistance to the use of healthcare as a way of oppressing fat

42 Meleo-Erwin, "Disrupting Normal: Toward the 'Ordinary and Familiar' in Fat Politics." This is echoed by Andrea Phillipson. Andrea Phillipson, "Re-Reading 'Lipoliteracy': Putting Emotions to Work in Fat Studies Scholarship," *Fat Studies: An Interdisciplinary Journal of Body Weight and Society* 2, no. 1 (2013): 70-86.

43 Guthman and DuPuis, "Embodying Neoliberalism: Economy, Culture, and the Politics of Fat."

44 And some are, for example the work being done within the critical dietetics community seeks to reinstate a political and social consciousness to HAES. Aphramor et al, "Critical Dietetics: A Declaration"; Jennifer Bradya et al, "Theorizing Health at Every Size as a Relational–Cultural Endeavour," *Critical Public Health* 23, no. 3 (2013): 345–55. See also Michelle Allison's blog, Michelle Allison, "The Fat Nutritionist," http://www.fatnutritionist.com/. May Friedman's important paper on fat activism and social work is relevant here too as an opportunity for professionals to rethink their fatphobia. May Friedman, "Fat Is a Social Work Issue: Fat Bodies, Moral Regulation, and the History of Social Work," *Intersectionalities: A Global Journal of 2012 Social Work Analysis, Research, Polity, and Practice* 1 (2012): 53-69.

people, and so of course this is what we're talking about since this is the purview, and we're trying to basically say, "We're not going to use BMI [Body Mass Index] as a proxy for health," but then we're still healthcare providers and so we are going to say, "But we do have to have some idea of what we're talking about when we're, or what we're supporting, if it's not going to be BMI what's it going to be?" and so we end up talking a lot about health and that keeps us very centred in this sometimes uncritical acceptance of the importance of health as a means of according someone worth, which is the healthism problem. (Eve)

Healthist fat activism downplays important connections with disability politics because it does not regard disability, ill health or impairment as part of the project of becoming good citizens. Disability and health overlap, intermingle and come and go in various ways. A large constituency of fat people are disabled and experience impairment and on-going encounters with medical institutions. I have written extensively elsewhere about the intimate connections between fat and disability.[45] Yet healthism in fat activism precludes the development of rich alliances between fat and disabled people,[46] including acknowledgment and understanding of ill health or impairment, in favour of a bland foreclosure of what people and bodies can and should be. It impedes critical connections with medicalisation or pathology as political systems or the possibility of queering fat and disability.[47] The healthist gentrification of fat activism reinforces a divide between good and bad fat people.

45 Charlotte Cooper, "Can a Fat Woman Call Herself Disabled?" *Disability & Society* 12, no. 1 (Feb 1997): 31-41; Cooper, *Fat & Proud*.
46 Although some scholars are highly engaged with these themes. April Herndon, "Disparate but Disabled: Fat Embodiment and Disability Studies," *National Women's Studies Association Journal* 14, no. 3 (2002): 121-37; Amber Cantrell, "Freaking Fatness through History: Critical Intersections of Fatness and Disability," *Chrestomathy: Annual Review of Undergraduate Research* 12 (2013): 1-39; Anna Mollow, "Disability Studies Gets Fat," *Hypatia* 30, no. 1 (2015): 199-216.
47 Robert McRuer, *Crip Theory: Cultural Signs of Queerness and Disability* (New York: New York University Press, 2006).

RETHINKING BORDERS

Another way of talking about neoliberal fat activist access is assimilation, which means identifying with dominant culture and wanting to be a part of it. LeBesco sees fat activism as split between assimilationist and liberationist tendencies.[48] One is transgressive, it "revolts," and the other upholds normativity. LeBesco associates assimilationist fat activism with the consumerism of fatshion, for example she argues that "fat folk are embraced as consuming subjects but not as social subjects".[49] But in outfit-blogging, for example, they might assume both roles, consumer and activist overlap and are not mutually exclusive. Like LeBesco, I want to encourage fat activists to think about the contexts in which activism takes place. Some fat activism is revolutionary and some is not. But the distinction between liberationist and assimilationist fat activism is not always very clear.

For example, it is not enough to dismiss an intervention like a plus size clothes shop as a neoliberal space of little value to the bigger work of social change. Between November 2008 and 2011 Re/Dress NYC was a shop in Brooklyn selling new and second hand plus-size clothing. As a capitalist and consumerist enterprise, profit was the bottom line and, when a shop was no longer financially viable, it shed its overheads, including a staff of several people, and moved online. This is typical of other plus-size clothing retailers, both corporate and local. However, Re/Dress NYC was owned by Deb Malkin, who has a background in fat queer community organising, including the Fat Girl Flea Market, NOLOSE and various fundraisers. As well as being a shop, the Re/Dress NYC site in Brooklyn was also a community hub, a performance space, and hosted benefits for people in need. The people who worked and shopped at Re/Dress NYC also participated within other activist networks. Re/Dress NYC could be seen as a hybrid for-profit appropriation of a social enterprise model, where community involvement is regarded as good for business and vice

48 LeBesco, *Revolting Bodies*.
49 LeBesco, *Revolting Bodies*, 70.

versa. This is thoroughly located in US consumerism and neoliberalism, where access to money influences one's access to community, and where community space is sacrificed when the economy fails. These factors are indeed problematic and do raise questions about the implications of locating activism within consumerism. However, a place like Re/Dress cannot be considered a mono-dimensional entity, particularly given the pleasure and kinship that people experienced in the space.

The following exchange with Adiva, talking about the differences between NAAFA and NOLOSE, reiterates how difficult it is to distinguish between assimilationist and liberationist fat activism.

> I think that a conference like NAAFA does not feel like a queer conference to me, even though there are queer people on the board, and queer workshops, I've led a queer workshop there, it doesn't feel queer even though there are people at NAAFA and people at NOLOSE who are the same people. I don't really, I don't actually fully understand that but I know that having that queerness, just feeling like, it's almost like a love of just fucking things up, and like fucking with stuff. It's so important. It's like beyond this identification. What do you think? Tell me.

> Charlotte: Ok, what I think is queer fat activism is the edge, the edge of it, it's not to be assimilationist, whereas something like NAAFA, which represents a very straight view of fat activism to me, is about trying to get a seat at the master's table. I think queer fat activism is about kicking the table over and shitting all over it.

> Yeah, and you know I think that that feels as though it should be the right answer, but when I look at all of the politics of what happens at NAAFA and at NOLOSE, NAAFA's a lot more radical in some ways. So I mean NAAFA is a place where supersized people, or superfat people can be, and NOLOSE, I mean I almost didn't go back to NOLOSE because it was so not that.

Charlotte: Yes, maybe I'm using NAAFA as a shorthand for something else.

Yes, I totally agree and I think it's not that easy because I think there are ways that our queer spaces are very [political?]. I mean lots of weight loss surgery in the NOLOSE community, which is not at all kicking over the master's table, so I agree it has that feeling, but I don't know how to articulate the difference. (Adiva)

This conversation demonstrates that categories of place and activist style cannot be assumed, they can be read and experienced in different ways.

Being a fat activist is sometimes a vile, lonely and depressing experience, I am a part of a movement that can be alienating and oppressive and this must change if it is to be truly socially transformative. But dominant and problematic forms of fat activism are unlikely to disappear because, whilst neoliberalism continues, the movement will reflect and be constituted by its values. Queer and feminist fat activist space cannot be universally taken for granted as revolutionary, for example, and spaces presumed to be assimilationist or conservative might also maintain some capacity for transgression. Activism that is limited or problematic is still activism. The tactics and concepts available to the majority of fat activists are frequently imperfect or inadequate yet they are nevertheless experienced by them as a positive endeavour. It is the multiplicity of fat activism that is important to preserve and develop, its broadness is its power. In writing about these tensions my aim is to stop them being taken for granted as the only possible direction for fat activism, and to develop more socially conscious social change. Yet I acknowledge that interrogating and critiquing junk fat activism is a delicate business precisely because of the contradictions, ambiguities and ambivalences within it. These might be read as queer, which I shall now discuss.

QUEERING

I have explored what I think fat activism isn't and what I think it is. I have proposed other ways of finding out and knowing about fat activism. I have offered some ideas for contextualising and historicising parts of the movement and I have discussed some of the problems that occur when the dynamism of radical fat activist ethics are put aside. Right now fat activism is at a crossroads. This critical juncture represents a choice to continue sleepwalking through a neoliberal social movement, to maintain an investment in proxies for fat activism, or to find other directions.

In this final chapter I want to present some of the strategies and styles of fat activism that I think offer ways of addressing the tensions that are currently hindering it as a social movement, for example by making space for the weird or indefinable, and reconnecting with the values of earlier activism. To do this, I will present four queer fat feminist projects that I originated and developed in the UK in recent years, which make use of queer theory.

DEFINING QUEER

Queer means different things to different people but I am using it here to describe both a sexual identity and a quality.

More inclusive than the binary categories of lesbian and gay, queer encompasses other non-heteronormative sexualities and genders. Queer is a way of saying that identity is socially constructed.[1] Judith Butler describes queer as an anti-identity because its constituency is so extensive and indefinable.[2] It recognises the unfixed nature of sexual desire and gender expression, it reflects what one *does* rather than who one *is*.[3] Queer rhymes with sneer and has an anti-normative, anti-assimilationist and punk streak to it. Yet in some circles queer contradicts this and has also become a synonym for a restrictive kind of gay identity, that of young, able-bodied, white, affluent, conformist, urban men.[4] This paradox illustrates the slippery nature of queer and the difficulty, or rather inappropriateness, of trying to pin it down. Queering fat activism involves acknowledging the foundational presence and contributions of queers to the movement. It is fat activism done by queers.[5]

In addition, queer is a sensibility that can influence action. To queer fat activism also means bringing particular qualities to it. Noreen Giffney's take on queer offers a sense of openness and possibility.

> There is an unremitting emphasis in queer theoretical work on fluidity, über-inclusivity, indeterminacy, indefinibility, unknowability, the preposterous, impossibility, unthinkability, unintelligibility, meaninglessness and that which is unrepresentable and uncommunicable. [...] There is an underlying belief permeating the field that some things cannot be explained and that is okay. In this, queer theory seeks to allow for complexity and the holding of uncertaincies by encouraging the experiencing of states without necessarily trying to understand, dissect or categorise them.[6]

1 Foucault, *The History of Sexuality, Vol. 1*.

2 Judith Butler, *Gender Trouble: Feminism and the Subversion of Identity* (New York: Routledge, 2006).

3 Jagose, *Queer Theory*.

4 David L. Eng et al, "What's Queer About Queer Studies Now?" *Social Text* 23, no. 3-4 (2005): 1-17.

5 Cat Pausé et al eds, *Queering Fat Embodiment* (Farnham: Ashgate, 2014).

6 Noreen Giffney, "Introduction: The 'Q' Word" in *The Ashgate Research Companion to Queer Theory*, edited by Noreen Giffney and Michael O'Rourke, 1-13 (Farnham: Ashgate Publishing Ltd, 2009).

I find this evocation of queer helpful in thinking through the aspects of fat activism that do not conform to an idea of purpose, unity, progress, the rational or the upstanding. It is a fat activism that does not need to be defined through dominant culture. I have often cringed at the idea that fat activism is not real or effective, that it is a joke. But Giffney's inclusion of the preposterous here gives activists permission to go off in their own way and not to worry too much about propriety. As queer loosens up how people think of identity, it also unfixes ideas about what the movement or fat activism can be.

To queer is to connect with that which is subversive and breaks rules.[7] Zoë Meleo-Erwin argues that queering moves fat people beyond a discourse of shame to reclaim the messy, disobedient aspects of ourselves.[8] Kris noted:

> It's celebrating the hideousness of the margins or whatever it is that has left us out, made us the last-picked, made us feel alone and sad and unworthy and all the negative things of fatness and queerness and gender etc, and race [...]. When people do find voice from those places it's really incredible and life-changing. (Kris)

To queer fat activism is also to relinquish the desire to be normal, respectable and polite. It entails identifying with the Other. Daniah recalled their own process of moving from trying to present themselves as upright, healthist subjects in their performance practice to developing work that no longer upheld those values:

> And so then our performance started to change, especially as we went to NOLOSE. And we decided that we didn't really give a fuck about trying to show everyone that our bodies were the

7 Judith Halberstam, "The Anti-Social Turn in Queer Studies," *Graduate Journal of Social Science* 5, no. 2 (2008): 140-56.
8 Zoë Meleo-Erwin, "Queering the Linkages and Divergences: The Relationship between Fatness and Disability and the Hope for a Livable World" in *Queering Fat Embodiment*, edited by Cat Pausé et al, 97-114 (Farnham: Ashgate, 2014).

same as [theirs], because we didn't really know what that meant any more, whose bodies we wanted to show that ours were the same as, because we already gave much more fat pride and didn't care about showing people that we could do the splits or whatever. So then we started playing more with food and sex and you know, doing much more gruesome style of performances. For example in one of our performances we basically built a gigantic ice cream sundae, then we pretended to fuck the ice cream, fuck each other, we rolled around, we were covered in ice cream, and we were crazy. (Daniah)

To queer fat is to enjoy its recalcitrance. Julia described the delight of being queerly anti-social in her joyful account of watching the fat and queer singer Beth Ditto in action.

I kind of connected to her on a level, totally, and in terms of how punk it is to just be a fat naked person on stage and be, "I don't give a fuck and I also don't shave and I don't wear deodorant and I'm completely comfortable with my physicality and I don't care whether it shocks you," how incredible that was, and how much more that spoke to me than, because, you know, I've always been into punk, but how much more that spoke to me than, like, skinny white boys trashing their guitars and things like that. No, this is much better! And I heard a story of when she was getting fatphobic comments at, I think, a gig in Australia or something, that she totally took them to task and made herself vomit on the stage [Charlotte laughs] which I thought was fantastic. (Julia)

Queer theory has a reputation for being incorporeal and highly abstract, but queering fat activism entails an appreciation of uncontained and lawless embodiment. As Hannah put it:

The most exciting thing about fat queers is their aggressive embodiment. Like, I'm so excited when I meet any fat queers

who are large and in charge in their bodies and in themselves, and
are taking up space in the world. I think for me that's the most
fundamental kind of amazing activism, like in refusing to die, and
taking up as much space as possible. (Hannah)

Queer can apply to all of the other forms of fat activism I mentioned
in earlier chapters, not just that which is ambiguous, although it can
certainly make sense of that. I will give examples later on where queer
has been brought to community-building, cultural production and micro
activism. It can also be a part of political process activism. For example,
at the March for the Alternative, an anti-Austerity demonstration in
London organised by the Trades Union Congress on 26 March 2011, a
small group of us participated as the FAT BLOC.[9] This was a reference to
the use of Black Blocs by anarchists at protests, which had been adapted
to Pink Blocs and Glitter Blocs by queer anarchist protesters through
non-violent tactical frivolity. We made a big, glittery, rainbow FAT BLOC
placard and took part. In retrospect it is clear to me that Austerity is a
policy that has been used to attack fat people, especially those who are
also poor and disabled, for example through arguing that we cost the
state too much money to support.[10] But in 2011 these positions were not
widely known. We took the decision to be a FAT BLOC because we felt
that the Left needed to recognise the presence of fat queer anarchists and
we wanted to have a bit of a laugh. This entailed some not entirely jokey
interactions with people using "fat cat" and fat capitalist symbolism on
their own placards, asking them to think about their use of fat stereotypes,
especially concerning class, and to support fat queers! Street protests and
unions are classic forms of political process activism and here we were

9 The "A" in FAT being an anarchist "circled A" symbol.

10 In 2015 The British Government announced that they were researching ways of
sanctioning fat people on benefits who refused treatment. Carol Black, "An Independent
Review into the Impact on Employment Outcomes of Drug or Alcohol Addiction,
and Obesity," edited by Department for Work and Pensions (London: Government
of the United Kingdon, 2015). See also Stinson's comments about the effects of such
sanctions. Stinson, "Nothing Succeeds Like Excess".

gleefully queering them.

In the previous chapter I discussed some of the problems that arise in the movement when boundary-keeping is enforced. But queering fat activism involves regarding difficult conversations, inclusion of undesirables and the breaking down of boundaries as helpful things to do. It is complexity rather than simplicity that is sought. This version of queer is not the postmodern fragmentation of social justice activism feared by some social movement theorists, instead it is about expanding activism and encouraging people to recognise their agency and participation. Noreen Giffney and Michael O'Rourke propose that queer opens up closed binary categories and enables new and hybrid spaces to flourish.[11] As Kerry pointed out:

> [...] what you realise about non-normativity is that it's a much bigger constituency than normativity because normativity very quickly emerges as a myth and a fiction. (Kerry)

To LeBesco, a queered fat activism is one based on the affinities of diverse people rather than organisations built on shared identities.

> What I find most compelling about this is the move away from organisation based on shared essential traits, towards affinities of action. While there is still some identity-based core, the new emphasis is on working with others to achieve similar goals.[12]

But I would argue that even here the idea of shared goals alludes to a valuing of sameness to some extent. Instead of, or as well as this, queering fat activism could be about creating a non-conformist social movement where there is space for people to be different to each other and for

---

11 Noreen Giffney and Michael O'Rourke, *The Ashgate Research Companion to Queer Theory* (Farnham: Ashgate Publishing Ltd, 2009).
12 LeBesco, *Revolting Bodies*.

things to emerge from that difference.[13] Liz illustrated this when she stated that she doesn't need other people to be the same as her in order to form activist alliances:

> I live in this plus-size fashion world, also I am waaay radical for a lot of people, and I, you know, and I choose to engage in certain ways. But if I had a litmus test I wouldn't have any colleagues or friends, except for maybe one person I can think of. And I don't want to have that, and I don't actually expect most people to believe what I believe, I really don't, and I don't need them to. But like, and I think because I don't need them to, we can be in the same space together. (Liz)

Liz' point of view is evident in the examples I will share below, where people who would not normally have been positioned as fat activists were invited to take part, or volunteered themselves as participants. I see this not as the evangelism and outreach of political process fat activism, I am not interested in converting people to my point of view in these projects. Instead I see this as a queer tactic of disrupting false binaries and unhelpful boundary-making so that people can come together and be different simultaneously.

Whilst there is generally a paucity of theorising within fat activism, some queer theorists have attempted to apply queer to fat activism, although the authors' engagement with the movement tends to be limited and the works are usually intended for an academic readership. Michael Moon and Eve Kosofsky Sedgwick were perhaps the first to have a go at queering fat. They argue that as queer is a defiant reclaiming of a concept that has been used to threaten and disgust, so fat activists might also set about reclaiming their own perceived wretchedness as a source of strength.[14] LeBesco develops this idea, playing on the term 'revolting',

13 Linnell Secomb, "Fractured Community," *Hypatia* 15, no. 2 (2000): 133-50.
14 Moon's speculation is loaded with errors but he also recognises that queering fat can support new methods of understanding the subject. His discussion with Kosofsky Sedgwick acknowledges that this is not going to come out of obesity discourse. Michael

noting fat bodies are positioned as revolting, as in repellent. But she notes
that there is a double meaning of revolting, which she envisages as fully
embodied resistance and an important source of power.[15] A different way
of putting this is through the term resignifying meaning that "we just
might be able to talk our way out of anything, even seemingly entrenched
fat oppression".[16] But Samantha Murray dismisses this claim, arguing that,
because fat embodiment is undeniable, fat activism is a futile endeavour
of "overcoming the body" and that attempts to resignify fat abjection,
through performance for example, merely reproduce it.[17] Whether or not
fat activism resignifies fat is perhaps not the issue. Queer theory would
allow for both: resignification may be possible through fat activism in
some instances and not others, depending on the context. More recently
queer has resurfaced as a means of exploring intersections of identity
and normativity concerning fat, particularly through the idea of the
death drive.[18] In an edited collection about the influence of Georges
Bataille,[19] Lynne Gerber proposes that the move towards respectability
in fat activism should be replaced with a more tolerant exploration of the
gross, queer excess inherent to the social construction of fat in the West.[20]
Through a discussion of the performer Divine, Susan Stinson's fiction and
FaT GiRL, she invites fat activists to consider how queer constructions

Moon and Eve Kosofsky Sedgwick, "Divinity: A Dossier, a Performance Piece, a
Little-Understood Emotion" in *Tendencies*, edited by Eve Kosofsky Sedgwick, 211-46
(Durham, NC: Duke University Press, 1994).

15 Kathleen LeBesco, "Queering Fat Bodies/Politics" in *Bodies out of Bounds: Fatness
and Transgression*, edited by J.E. Braziel and Kathleen LeBesco, 74-87 (Los Angeles:
University of California Press, 2001). There are some contradictions in her theory, for
example treating fat as innately queer looks like another form of essentialism. Of course
this might not matter, queer is a means of accommodating contradictions.

16 LeBesco, "Queering Fat Bodies/Politics," 77.

17 Murray, *The 'Fat' Female Body*. Murray's argument here is not convincing, fat
activist literature includes many references to embodiment, not "overcoming the
body." She makes some unsubstantiated claims, for example, it is not true that Pretty
Porky and Pissed-Off performed only to fat audiences, as she states. This undermines
the reliability of the text.

18 A psychoanalytic theory about self-destruction.

19 A French philosopher interested in transgressive sex.

20 Gerber, "Movements of Luxurious Exuberence."

of death might offer a means of experiencing fat more compassionately. By limiting her analysis to interventions based in the US, Gerber misses Francis Ray White's essay, which has already responded to her proposal in actual activist terms. In their discussion of the death drive in queer theory, White uses The Chubsters, of which more later, to describe how fat activists might develop "a refusal of both more established fat politics and of reproductive futurism more generally"[21] to embrace freakhood and repudiate the crusade towards wholesome happiness in fat activism.

I realise that queer is contentious. This means that even where queer is an appropriate way of understanding something, people are reluctant to use it.[22] Resisting normativity is safer for some people than others because of privilege and access or lack of it. Like fat, queer is a concept around which many people feel threatened and its use requires people to address their homophobia. It is also commonly dismissed as too abstract, too preoccupied with high theory, as irrelevant to grassroots activism. I will show that these criticisms are more to do with theoretical snobbery because fat activists are already using queer in material ways.[23]

I would also like to add a note of caution. Whilst queered fat activism

---

21 Francis Ray White, "Fat, Queer, Dead: 'Obesity' and the Death Drive," *Somatechnics* 2, no. 1 (2012): 1-17. Reproductive futurism refers to an idea of becoming normal through participating in the institutions of family and baby-making and therefore creating a future for humanity.

22 Elizabeth Armstrong and Mary Bernstein's "awkward social movements" look very queer, yet neither they nor other authors writing about poststructuralist social movements take up the challenge of applying it to their work. Armstrong and Bernstein, "Culture, Power, and Institutions."

23 Suzanna Danuta Walters, "From Here to Queer: Radical Feminism, Postmodernism, and the Lesbian Menace" in *Queer Theory*, edited by Iain Morland and Annabelle Willox, 6-21 (Basingstoke: Palgrave Macmillan, 2005); Tim Edwards, "Queer Fears: Against the Cultural Turn," *Sexualities* 1, no. 4 (1998): 471-84; Clarke, "Finding the Subject: Queering the Archive"; George Katsiaficas, "Reading Signs of Change: Social Movement Cultures 1960s to Now" in *Signs of Change*, edited by Dara Greenwald and Josh MacPhee, 16-21 (Oakland and New York: AK Press/Exit Art, 2010); Michael Warner, "Queer and Then? The End of Queer Theory?" *The Chronicle of Higher Education*, http://chronicle.com/article/QueerThen-/130161; Jack Halberstam et al, "Bullybloggers on Failure and the Future of Queer Studies," *Bully Bloggers*, http://bullybloggers.wordpress.com/2012/04/02/bullybloggers-on-failure-and-the-future-of-queer-studies/.

makes space for interventions that are context-specific or ambiguous, these should not be treated as superior to other types of action. I have argued against the dominance of some forms of fat activism over others and I am not advocating a replacement style that can now overtake other types of activism. Activists should beware of creating a fundamentalist movement, a return to an imagined purer past, new orthodoxies, or a replacement monoculture. It is not enough to substitute one set of assumptions about fat activism with another. More traditional models for social change, such as rights-based activism, remain vital. Benjamin's account of witnessing a speech exemplified this pluralism well:

> I just remember being at that NOLOSE when Lynn McAfee talked, and just bawling my eyes out, and oh it isn't all about fucking and, like, being punk and, like, having sex. It is about rights, and there are people actually who are, and it is important, I'm the person at the cabaret and doing the dance party and wearing tight pants. But there's actually someone trying to advocate for me somewhere, and we have to nod our head to that and hope that that person's a homo but it probably doesn't matter, you know what I mean?! (Benjamin)

QUEER FAT ACTIVISM

During the course of the research for this book I developed a series of interrelated projects where queer people and Giffney's queer qualities were central. They are not the only kinds of fat activism that I have done or do. Like many fat activists my activism strays more towards cultural and micro forms and I continue to do this because, as I have stated, I think that many approaches are needed to create social change. I am not offering these examples as a blueprint for queer fat activism. They are contextual autoethnographic examples of what might happen when activists embrace queer. These projects illustrate how queer theory could be used by activists in practise, they move it out of the ivory tower, from abstraction to the concrete, and reinvigorate it with the energy of everyday people and everyday life.

These projects were a girl gang, a harvest festival, a way of recording and thinking about history, and an Olympics. The first pre-existed the research study and the others emerged indirectly from it between 2009 and 2012 as I began to become more interested in the application of queer theory to fat activism and activism in general. What they have in common is that they represented an explosion of options,[24] they were platforms from which many things could emerge, they were expansive yet also composed of smaller acts, some of which had been repeated elsewhere.[25] They included people of all sizes without constructing thinner people as allies, an assumption was made that everyone involved had a relationship to fat activism and that differences in relating are to be expected. They made use of online spaces as archives and promotional tools, and most of these projects have a theme song. The Chubsters, The Fat of the Land, *A Queer and Trans Fat Activist Timeline* and The Fattylympics were examples of fat activism where the imagination ran riot and where ambiguity was treated as an asset. They could afford to be experimental because they were cheap, mostly self-funded and independent, happy to be amateur. Most of these projects were part of a fat activist genealogy of the ridiculous founded in 1967 by the Fat-In and present in some of the Fat Underground's zaps. Sometimes these projects used anti-social aesthetics, but they were always rooted in social justice. They took fat people's right to exist for granted and were not a plea for understanding.

THE CHUBSTERS

The Chubsters began as a silly idea but developed into a model for doing fat activism that I was able to apply elsewhere. It became my prototype

---

24 Thanks to Ann Kaloski Naylor for this observation.
25 See, for example, my account of spitting on the BMI chart. Charlotte Cooper, "Hey Sisters, Welcome to My World" in *Hot & Heavy: Fierce Fat Girls on Life, Love and Fashion*, edited by Virgie Tovar, 65-70 (Berkeley, CA: Seal Press, 2012).

for fat activism that played with identity politics, humour, imagination and a sense of the unreal, the anti-social, and multi-directional activities.

The project was formulated as a queer fat girl gang I established in 2003 after watching Katrina Del Mar's low budget short film *Gang Girls 2000*, which created an imaginary world of queer gangs in New York.[26] I imagined The Chubsters as existing in a similar universe where fat people take no shit and I hoped that this could bleed into real life. I enjoyed the blurring of fiction and reality. I used the gang to play with ideas of comic aggression and anti-social behaviour yet was explicit in my pacifism and welcomed all to take part; Chubsters did not have to be fat, queer, a girl or even remotely vicious. On reflection I suspect this approach stemmed from my own experiences of queer exclusion from lesbian feminist spaces in the 1980s.

The Chubsters operated through a website, a magazine photo-story, articles, workshops, talks and film-shows, a theme song, a short film and objects and ideas. These included a symbol, called The Screaming C, a snarling fat letter C with blood-dripping fangs, designed by two Chubsters, Yeti and Big Blu in 2004. The symbol became a useful manifestation of the gang.[27] Other people adopted it, one person made me a hoodie decorated with The Screaming C, another is a stonemason and carved it into a plaque. In addition, The Chubsters produced hand signs, special terminology,[28] a call and response; downloads for calling cards; and gang colours stitched onto torn denim waistcoats and worn in public. Another member made some Chubster embroidery. The project

---

26 Charlotte Cooper, "The Chubsters," http://charlottecooper.net/b/chubsters/; Charlotte Cooper, "Chubsters Vs Imps," *Cheap Date*, 2005, 16-20; Charlotte Cooper, "The Story of the Chubsters" in *Pop Culture Association/American Culture Association*, edited by L. Owen and J. McCrossin (Marriott, New Orleans, 2009); Ines Voigts et al, "The Chubsters: Interview Mit Charlotte Cooper," *Hugs and Kisses: tender to all gender* no. 5 (15 October 2009): 52-55; Ines Voigts and Claus Gesine, "Invasion of the Chubsters," *an.schläge*, December/January (2010): 20-21.

27 There have been Screaming Cs on walls and hoardings around London at various times. Some of us drew one into some wet concrete on the street where I live and it is still there, years later. I also have a tattoo of the Screaming C on my hip, as does Chubster Butch Husky. Today I graffitied it on a door.

28 Narrow Fucks, for example, meaning narrow-minded fatphobes.

sprawled all over the place, I did not try to control this because I enjoyed the random strangeness that the idea sparked in people.

The gang existed in real spaces but its power was in the way it used the immaterial and the imagination. It enabled people to conceptualise fat people as brilliant, creative, nonsensical, eye-popping, sublime, intimidating, strong and as a group that cared for each other and welcomed sympathisers. As a gang, The Chubsters valued anti-social unruliness; we did not want to be nice, respectable girls. We revelled in the margins. This was a powerful experience for many of those who encountered the project because, in the early days of obesity epidemic rhetoric around 2000, the idea of fat as utterly worthless had become widespread. The Chubsters deflated the pomposity of that rhetoric by treating it as unimportant. We refused to be drawn to the debate being instilled because it did not reflect our reality, an important queer tactic. Rather than being intelligible to agents of power it was more important to speak to and recognise each other on our own terms and to make our own culture, no matter how bizarre. Besides, we had an arsenal of spud guns[29] and plenty of members with itchy trigger fingers.

Queer and fat embodiment was important in The Chubsters. Members would encourage each other to be daring and wild, and to enjoy the forbidden thrills of being fat. In workshops extraordinary scenes would unfold, for example the superfat Apple Hard turned a cartwheel, El-Assessino did astonishing martial arts kicking, spontaneous dancing would break out, a mass group of fat queers simultaneously belly-smashed an initiate. Chubster embodiment was happily grotesque. Spitting, wobbling, sneering, glaring were acts employed to undermine the worship of normativity within obesity discourse.

At its height The Chubsters had over 100 members, though I often lied about this and implied that there were many more. I didn't think being a member mattered, but I thought people might like having a badge

---

29 Toy guns that shoot pellets of potato with compressed air. A satirical and non-violent nod to the question of whether or not activists should bear arms, and also the carbohydrate ruination of dieters.

and a card. To become a member involved asking to join via email or attending a workshop where people would be jumped-in. This usually meant shouting and group belly-smashes. For some time I stipulated that prospective members do something Chubster-worthy, but people were either too intimidated to act or did things for which I did not want to be responsible, so that requirement ended. New members were given a badge, a membership card with a drawing of their face, and they would be encouraged to invent a persona and have a profile on the website. No money changed hands, I paid for badges, postage and web space myself, a negligible amount. When a beloved fat activist and Chubster Heather MacAllister, aka Beelzebubba, died in 2007, her membership card was returned to me by her partner for safe-keeping.

The Chubsters became something I talked about rather than actively pursued around 2010. When a second Chubster died in tragic circumstances I felt too sad to go on.[30] Social media was also changing, my web development skills were limited and the website remained rather static. I left it up for a while and then took it down. But the main problem was that as it became more popular, fat activists from the US started expecting the group to operate like a democratic organisation, as if that was the only way that the world of the Chubster imagination could be made real or useful. They were disappointed that I didn't use the gang to pursue political process goals, they thought that the project would only be worthwhile if it was as serious and focussed as they imagined activism to be. On the one hand these responses enabled me to think about the pigeonholing of fat activism and when interviewed about the gang I would make up fictitious stories for journalists as a strategy for handling their inevitable misrecognition. But on the other it seemed unbearably restrictive, I was being pressured into conforming to a dominant mode of activism in order to be legible to other people in the US and not for the first time.[31] This felt oppressive, I was expected to do what I was

30 The beautiful Frito Lay, also known as Elizabeth "Luscious" Baxter.
31 During its lifetime The Chubsters was misread as a support group, an anti-stigma organisation, an insult to the misery of gang culture in the USA, a prompt to commit vandalism, an exclusive clique for cool people.

told and I felt unable to handle other people's need for propriety. The outcome might have been different if the critics had come forward to act, but those who proposed projects never followed them through and emails I sent remained unanswered.

THE FAT OF THE LAND: A QUEER CHUB HARVEST FESTIVAL

In 2009 NOLOSE made small amounts of funding available for fat queer community development projects. At the time, and probably because of my experiences with The Chubsters, I was interested in trying to strengthen international bonds with fat queer organisations in the US, challenge what I felt was their parochialism, and gain recognition there for fat activism elsewhere. I applied for and was awarded a loan of about £600 or $1000.

The Fat of The Land was an event that used a queered and secular harvest festival as a celebration of abundance. It began as idea developed with my friend Jason Barker, we thought that a harvest festival would be a ludicrous format for a queer and trans fat gathering, but also one with a local flavour that was also relevant to people of many cultures. We invited Nazmia Jamal to be a co-organiser. The three of us knew each other from queer and DIY culture in London and we came from different activist traditions.[32] Not all of us identified as fat.

The event took place on 3 October 2009 at St Anne's, a gay-friendly church hall in Soho, London's mainstream gay village, to coincide with that year's Harvest Moon. The church setting was part of the event's theatricality rather than a reflection of any religious values. There were performances by poets and women Morris Dancers, I wrote and taught participants "The Fat Queer Harvest Hymn" which we then sang together, there were games and stalls, Nazmia curated an art installation of Allyson

32 As I write this, I am wondering if the immersive performances developed by Duckie in London's queer club scene influenced our decision to create this event. Catherine Silverstone, "Duckie's Gay Shame: Critiquing Pride and Selling Shame in Club Performance," *Contemporary Theatre Review* 22, no. 1 (2012): 62-78.

Mitchell's work, there was a raffle and traditional competitions for best cakes, jams and so on. As with the Chubsters, The Fat of The Land encouraged people to make things along the theme, using whatever skills they had. Some of these ended up as raffle prizes, for example some art by Lady Lucy, and others became objects in their own right, for example Simon Murphy made an electronic wire buzzer game of the word 'Chubster'. Thomas Appleton gave a display of his stonemasonry. I blogged the process of the project so that there would be an online archive of it and also to build interest in the event.[33]

With The Fat of The Land, building an intersectional community space on the basis of this difference meant inviting people who had little concept of fat activism to be part of the event, as organisers and makers, to be central to it. This expanded the number of participants massively and made the event very popular,[34] but it also affected how far it was able to go in terms of creating a radical fat, queer and trans space. Many of the participants were deeply ambivalent about fat and there was nowhere for these feelings to be expressed in a helpful manner. The event satisfied the harvest festival format by queering it but the fat activist elements were sometimes pushed aside. In retrospect, The Fat of The Land exemplified the limitations of body positive fat activism; cupcakes can only go so far in soothing a culture of rampant fatphobia. Because food justice and HAES were the foundations for The Fat of The Land, the event did not destabilise health as the governing discourse of fat and upheld individualistic notions of well-being as a matter of food choices and physical jerks. It lacked the gorgeous and life-affirming mayhem and belligerence of The Chubsters, it was an activism of tea and chatting rather than the glorification of Satanic bitches. This meant that moments of fat abjection, the reading of a poem about a tragic fat person

33 Charlotte Cooper et al, "The Fat of the Land: A Queer Chub Harvest Festival" in *The Fat of the Land: A Queer Chub Harvest Festival*, edited by Charlotte Cooper, London, 2009.
34 Just as well! Everything was orientated towards paying back the loan which ultimately made the event very stressful to produce. I regretted the extent to which people were asked to pay for things, I prefer activism where participation is free.

for example, were awkward and horrifying and could not be queerly transformed into something more relatable. I was also complicit with these attempts to make the event tame. For example, I asked the artist Cathy Ward, whose work with gothic and occult-looking corn dollies I admired, to contribute some pieces to decorate the hall. She made a series of sculptures overflowing with grotesque fat and ears of wheat: uncontainable fat. I did not use them because I thought they were ugly and might upset people, which, of course, was precisely the point of them!

A QUEER AND TRANS FAT ACTIVIST TIMELINE

Like The Chubsters, *A Queer and Trans Fat Activist Timeline* started off as one thing and became lots of things. It was and is a queer history project that places queers and trans people at the centre whilst adopting a DIY approach to making history. It was less embodied than the other projects I have described in this section though it exists in material objects and is not entirely a cerebral exercise.

In 2010 I was actively seeking out archival holdings of fat activism and was inspired by what I had found. I wanted to record some histories of fat activism but to do this collectively and focus on ordinary people's memories and contributions to the movement. In 2003 I had been an oral history worker on a project by and about LGBT elders in the UK and my experiences there informed the kinds of material I was hoping to generate.[35] I was interested in how fat activist histories might be transmitted through communities because I was dismayed by how little fat activists seemed to know about the movement of which they were a part. I also felt that fat activism is under-documented and wanted to create a paper trail for others to use.

I proposed a workshop at that year's NOLOSE in Oakland and this was accepted. I knew that there would be older and younger delegates

---

35 Gay & Lesbian Arts and Media, "Before Stonewall: A Lesbian, Gay, Bisexual and Transgendered Oral History," London, 2004.

at the conference and I hoped to stimulate some intergenerational dialogue. At the workshop, my co-facilitator Kay Hyatt and I attached a long sheet of paper to the wall and marked it off year by year. We invited workshop participants to populate the sheet with thoughts and memories that related to those years, writing directly onto it with felt-tipped pens. I was vague in my definition of fat activism, I wanted to see what people would write, what fat activism meant to them. Together we created a timeline that documented this group's histories of fat activism. I made a couple of audio recordings of people telling their stories but I am sorry to say that I later erased them accidentally. It was exciting to see conversations unfold as the *Timeline* took shape over the course of an hour or so. Participants clustered around the paper and wrote and drew their contributions. People sought clarification with each other and talked about things that they were simultaneously historicising. Old and young people worked together as equal contributors. It was as though past and present were meeting.

The *Timeline* was of a very specific time and place and represented a particular group of people: queer and trans workshop participants at NOLOSE. I drew attention to this specificity at the workshop and elsewhere to question the idea that there is a universal fat activist history and to show that histories are contextualised by their location. I wanted to create cross-cultural critical dialogue about what it is to document fat activism and what it means to construct and interpret fat activist histories. As I travelled over the next six months I took the *Timeline* to a series of fat activist gatherings for discussion in San Leandro, London and Berlin. The object that was co-created at the workshop mutated into an object that travelled, that taught and that enabled people to talk together about fat activism as well as its cultural and temporal specificities.

I wanted more people to be able to access the *Timeline*, so I made it into a paper zine and a digital zine that people could download and read from my website, including an audio version for people with visual impairments or anybody who wanted to listen to it.[36] I created the zine

36 Cooper, "A Queer and Trans Fat Activist Timeline - Zine Download."

at an artist's residency in Hamburg, at Villa Magdalena K, a feminist art project. I thought it would be good to do this work outside a US or British context in a city where people had already been supportive of fat activism. During the residency, the *Timeline* became something that was talked about in the house and I was interviewed about it for a local queer feminist radio show. I recorded it in photographs and through a short film. I used the proceeds from selling the paper zine to post copies of it to feminist, queer and zine archives around the world. I wrote a paper about the project for an academic journal.[37]

In April 2011, when the zine was complete, I donated the original *Timeline* to Bildwechsel. This is a queer, trans and feminist multimedia archive that has its headquarters in Hamburg. Bildwechsel had sponsored a Chubsters film show at the 2009 Lesbisch Schwule Filmtage. It was important to me to give the *Timeline* to an archive and not maintain private ownership of it, I wanted more people to have access to it. Donating the material acknowledged the public and private in activist lives, that is, that private actions have public resonance. I wanted to lodge the *Timeline* in a place where English was spoken but where it is not people's first language, and where queer, trans and feminist politics were a given. I hoped that this would help it to mutate as a cultural artefact whilst preserving its integrity. I wanted to show that it isn't enough just to export identity politics, that they don't always fit different contexts, and to encourage people within those other contexts to speak back. I thought this might disrupt my own role as a fat activist who moves between countries and who may be an agent of cultural imperialism.

Later, in 2013, I created another *Timeline* with Fat Positivity Belgium, a queer and feminist fat activist group. I had been invited by the group to talk about my activism and I wanted to use that opportunity to engage with the movement together. In Brussels there were fewer expectations about what fat activism looks like because the members of the group had less experience of fat activist community than many of the Oakland

---

37 Cooper, "A Queer and Trans Fat Activist Timeline: Queering Fat Activist Nationality and Cultural Imperialism."

participants, but they had a more mature approach to intersectionality and inclusion and the group was very mixed. The content of the Brussels *Timeline* was more personal than Oakland and there was considerable puzzlement about what might be written because of the strangeness of thinking about one's actions and experiences as historically important. After the workshop the *Timeline* was donated to the group for them to develop or ignore as they chose.

A *Queer and Trans Fat Activist Timeline* was not a rowdy project like the others I have described here, but it remains allied to a queer sensibility. It was based on an idea of history that is not concerned with facts but with fuzzy memory and community collaboration. The content of both the Oakland and Brussels *Timelines* is frequently ambiguous; they name things but there are few details; they are happily incomplete, what is there and not there is a product of forgetting as much as remembering; they are inconsistent and muddled. This all challenges the notion of there being a single, universal, truthful fat activist history. Instead of trying to create an activism that simplifies and reduces a discourse, the *Timeline* invites many forms of dialogue across a number of sites and is a project that emphasises complexity and specificity.

Where The Chubsters ended and The Fat of the Land and The Fattylympics, which I will discuss below, were events circumscribed by time, the *Timeline* is still live as an archival object at Bildwechsel, as something owned by Fat Positivity Belgium, or through zine holdings in archives elsewhere. It is still available to download. It could still be turned into something else now or in the distant future. It hasn't ended. It was of a place but has moved into many other places. As it became a series of moments and objects, so its intentions, sites and effects multiplied. It is now owned by many different people. The format could be adapted by other people thinking about generating fat activist histories.

THE FATTYLYMPICS

The Fattylympics took place in London on 7 July 2012, two weeks before the beginning of the Olympic Games.[38] This was an idea that had been percolating since 2007 when London was made host city for the Games.[39] I live in the area where the Olympic Park was built and I witnessed, over a period of years, the decimation of my community by the International Olympic Committee and its supporters. Organised by Kay Hyatt and myself, The Fattylympics was conceived of as a fat activist response to a number of problems that the Olympics caused or exacerbated such as: social cleansing; gentrification; militarisation; corporatisation; nationalism; surveillance; the increased harassment of homeless people, sex workers, black and Asian youth by the authorities; the use of the Olympics to promote anti-fat policy, especially towards young people; the rhetoric of winning at all costs. The event was funded through my share of the profits of the Fat of The Land, which were invested in The Big Bum Jumble, its main fundraiser.[40] It took place at Grassroots Community Centre in West Ham, two miles from the Olympic Park.

This was the most complex event that I had ever organised and it took over a year to put in place. There would be an opening and closing ceremony, a guest of honour, an anthem, torches, a parade. There would be a series of original events. There would be medals for everyone who wanted one. There would be food and stalls. The space would need to be community-based and accessible. It all needed to have a bold queer and fat feel to it, to be unassimilated.

Vikki Chalklin started the day with a participatory performance of a kitsch fat queer aerobics class. She led us in to the opening ceremony,

38 Charlotte Cooper, "Fattylympics," http://fattylympics.blogspot.co.uk/; Carolyn Smith, "Under the Radar: Fat Activism and the London 2012 Olympics, an Interview with Charlotte Cooper," http://www.gamesmonitor.org.uk/node/1647.

39 Charlotte Cooper, "Olympics/Uhlympics: Living in the Shadow of the Beast," *thirdspace* 9, no. 2 (2010).

40 Charlotte Cooper and Kay Hyatt, "Big Bum Jumble," http://www.bigbumjumble.blogspot.co.uk/.

which consisted of people clanging a metal sculpture that was situated close to the venue and a parade of torches that Cathy Ward had made.[41] Anybody who wanted to parade the torches could parade them, so this took some time. Participants were invited to make a mass show of disrespect in the direction of the Olympic Park, and people took the opportunity to give it the finger, jeer and moon it together. Our guest of honour, Erkan Mustafa, a local person who had played the iconic fat character Roland in the British children's TV show *Grange Hill*, cut a ribbon and made a speech.[42] We sang "The Fattylympics Anthem", composed by Verity Susman with lyrics I had written, twice because we liked it so much. Following this, there were four events, all of which emphasised ridiculousness, amateurishness, accessibility and non-competitiveness. The first was Rolling With Roland, which involved rolling down a grassy bank. The second was Twirling, by Corinna Tomrley and Becky Sanchez, who also created The Fattylympics Mascots called Egg'n'Spoon. They performed a twirling routine and then invited people to twirl together. The third, Spin-Off, was created by Simon Murphy and entailed wearing special hats and getting very dizzy. People were encouraged to take the idea and make something from it so, for example, Bethan Evans and Rachel Colls formed The Fat Geography Massive and set up a gym knicker blinging station with sequins and glitter, and Lindsay Starbuck had created street art. Other stalls sold the by now usual mixture of clothes, food and HAES. The final event of the day was a round of spitting on the BMI chart. For me, a Fattylympics highlight was when a participant felt moved to retrieve and empty her Moon Cup[43] on the chart, to horrified, delighted and amazed looks. Although children were welcome, this was the point at which onlookers realised that The Fattylympics was not a family fun day out. Hundreds of unique home-made medals were given out at the closing ceremony, a woman did some fire dancing, we sang the "Anthem" a few more times and music was

---

41 This time I didn't turn down her spectacular work.
42 Erkan asked only to be paid in carrot cake, his favourite.
43 A device for collecting menstrual blood worn inside the vagina.

provided by Rhythms of Resistance, an anti-capitalist percussion band.

I retained some of the organising principles of The Chubsters and The Fat of The Land. The Fattylympics was a basic idea from which unexpected things could sprawl; it was a hybrid space, a fake Olympics that sought to highlight a multitude of intersectional issues; it was ridiculous and serious, irreverent and rude, though accessible to people of all ages, free and open to everyone; it emphasised making things and embodiment; it merged the real and the fantasy; it was a spectacle and it was local. The Fattylympics, like The Chubsters, was a space for addressing things on our own terms, and generally from the margins. Because of its queerness, and because fat activism is commonly perceived as inconsequential, if it is perceived at all, The Fattylympics was not always legible to other anti-Olympics protesters or activists with whom we sought to make alliances. During the organising period we were snubbed by a number of groups whom we approached as potential participants and this was disappointing.

Several years later it is difficult to convey the frenzy surrounding the summer of 2012 in East London. Surface-to-air missiles had been installed on blocks of flats as an anti-terrorist measure; a large "Police Hub" including custodial cells was erected in a local park; special Parliamentary orders were put in place criminalising anti-Olympics activities such as democratic protest; Olympic Lanes were painted on the roads so that officials could enjoy privileged travel by excluding all other traffic; everywhere was an eruption of flag-waving and self-congratulation. It was very difficult to find a venue in our local area because a great deal of public space had been commandeered for the Olympics. Anything that seemed as though it might be protesting the Games was heavily policed. Local authorities in the Olympic boroughs would not support events that were critical of the Olympics. The only day on which we could hold The Fattylympics at our venue coincided with the annual LGBT Pride march in central London and this meant that many of the people who might otherwise have come to our event went there instead. The London Organising Committee of the Olympic and Paralympic Games were also meticulous in protecting their corporate sponsors who had paid a lot of money for exclusive rights to the brand.

They ruthlessly pursued local people and businesses who broke their rules, such as using the words and symbols they controlled. We had to be secretive and careful to avoid prosecution. Instead of placing other people at risk, Kay and I took responsibility for the event and worked with collaborators instead of producing it collectively. But the secrecy of The Fattylympics could not be maintained in this excitable climate. I had blogged the project carefully but a journalist friend of a friend cut and pasted my interview with Erkan and published it without my permission in a popular right-wing broadsheet newspaper.[44] From then on we were plagued by other journalists. We made no comment. We did our best to eject the press from the event but a journalist and a photographer from *The Daily Mail* did not disclose their presence. That newspaper published photographs of participants taken without their knowledge or consent and a story making fun of us.[45] A pair of Brazilian journalists admitted their presence to us and produced more sympathetic stories, perhaps because they saw what was happening in London as foreshadowing what would come to their country in 2016.[46]

As far as I can tell, in spite of media intrusion the many people who came to The Fattylympics had a great day. People still ask me if there is going to be another one and are disappointed when I say no. Around a

---

44 Following pressure from my union, they eventually took it down but they never admitted who stole it and they never paid me for using my work.

45 Jill Foster, "The Roly-Poly Olympics!" *Associated Newspapers*, http://www.dailymail. co.uk/news/article-2170666/Fattylympics-The-Roly-poly-Olympics-Contestants-WERE-game-laugh.html#ixzz20DL84C4t. *The Daily Mail* literally misrecognised us by captioning a photograph of Vikki Chalklin with my name. This was not a problem for me, Vikki is gorgeous, but it might be an example of all fat people looking the same to a fatphobic media. I am not singling out *The Daily Mail* for fat hatred. The paper reproduced my press release for The Big Bum Jumble word for word and gave it a sympathetic though slightly odd write-up (by trying to hang it on a "Size Zero" hook, the tabloid fat debate *du jour* in 2010). Both left and right-wing media in the UK is mixed in terms of its coverage of fat, the country's leading left-leaning paper is often highly fatphobic.

46 Terra, "Ator Será O Líder Da 'Fattylympics', Protesto Contra Os Jogos," *Terra Networks Brasil S.A.*, http://esportes.terra.com.br/jogos-olimpicos/londres-2012/ noticias/0,,OI5877012-EI19410,00-Ator+sera+o+lider+da+Fattylympics+protesto+ contra+os+Jogos.html.

couple of hundred people came, from all walks of life, including local kids who were playing in the park and who stopped by to grab a medal. Many more talked about it on social media. This is not a mass movement, but the quality of people's engagement was very high. It was an opposite land, a playground where the ugliness of the Olympics and all that it represented didn't matter for a while. The Fattylympics was complex, multi-layered, something that lots of different kinds of people could get their teeth into. Together we created a moment where the Chubsters universe that I had originally imagined around ten years earlier was finally real in my neighbourhood. I considered it proof that other ways of being were possible. It was feminist and queer fat activism that had helped to engender that feeling.

WHO KNOWS?

I continue to draw on fat queer feminist activism through my cultural work and make platforms from which things can develop. In 2010 I co-founded a band called Homosexual Death Drive which plays with queer death drive theory and obscenity through music, objects, videos, performances and the production of discomfort, feelings and memories. I was and am part of a dance project called *SWAGGA*, which started in 2014, working with Alexandrina Hemsley and Jamila Johnson-Small as Project O. In both of these pieces of work the anti-social is more pronounced than it was with The Fat of The Land, *A Queer and Trans Fat Activist Timeline* and The Fattylympics though it is less didactic and polemical because these are artistic projects, ambiguous and interpretable. They involve claiming space on stages where older fat dykes might not be expected to be, as well as finding our own sounds and movement. The aesthetic continues to be multi-directional and intersectional. I remain concerned with the intergenerational transmission of fat activism, of the activist potential for archiving the movement through projects like this, and so both have been documented online.[47]

Beyond this, what binds *SWAGGA* and Homosexual Death Drive, The Fattylympics, The Fat of The Land and The Chubsters, though not *A Queer and Trans Fat Activist Timeline*, is that they have all been degraded in various ways by struggles against normativity and aggressive misrecognition. My activism is now frequently concerned with avoiding those intrusions. This may look like separatism but it is not, I continue to engage with dominant culture including obesity discourse, it is impossible not to. But I feel most free as a fat activist when I am producing work on my own terms or collectively with other marginal people. I am sure I am not alone. This suggests that the self-determination of all people is central to activism and brings me back to my original concerns with this book, of who gets to know and speak about fat.

Fat activism is habitually overlooked, assumed and dismissed, even by people within the movement, which is outrageous given how powerful it can be. In this book I have tried to show what fat activism looks like as I understand it. I have talked about how knowledge about fat activism is produced and used and how this is political and contextualised by the time and place in which it emerges. I have also explained how easy it is to stifle knowledge about fat activism, and to use fat activism to sacrifice certain kinds of apparently unwelcome people, including the movement's founders, the very giants on whose shoulders we are all carried. I have argued in favour of resisting the stagnation that happens when people speak for fat activism without being engaged with it and when people use strategies that reproduce rather than dismantle inequality. As I draw *Fat Activism: A Radical Social Movement* to a close I urge you to reject the idea that fat activism is about following a prescribed set of rules, aims and activities and instead be excited about its limitless possibilities for social transformation. Appreciating this can enable you to customise what is important, to make activism that is meaningful and not something dictated, automatic or assumed. Knowing what fat activism is and where

47 See http://www.homosexualdeathdrive.com and http://charlottecooper.net/b/performance.

it comes from matters because it enables you to understand how activist decisions have wider social repercussions. I want to embolden you to recognise discourse and theory, to develop dynamic work that adds to the movement's historical, geographical and cultural locations. This involves creating work that acknowledges the many ways in which fat activism takes place and its many contexts, not isolated proxies. I want to encourage you to develop new activism which reinstates critical anti-oppressive politics, creates a body of rigorous knowledge and makes demands of researchers.

Fat hatred has been around for a long time, but it is 15 years since The World Health Organization's report on obesity was published and this accelerated fat hatred in the 21st century by propagating fat panic.[48] The august authors of this report recommended measuring and classifying fat people, defining us as a major social problem and trying to find proof that we are a terrible burden to society and do not deserve support. They sought our prevention and management through an idea of weight loss that they think is robust and viable. Their work remains massively influential.[49] Yet there is no doubt that fat activism based on the lived experience, cultures and histories of fat people, which incorporates anti-oppressive values, feminist and queer tactics is able to offer a richer and more sophisticated vision for understanding fat than the proponents of obesity who remain intent on ignoring or belittling us.

So how might people know about fat? Through a disease model or through rolling down a hill together? Through bariatric surgery or poetry? Through terrible clinical encounters or a fat clothes swap? Through weight loss drugs that cause heart attacks and anal leakage or by reading *Fat Liberator Publications*? Through Very Low Calorie Diets or by visiting

---

48 World Health Organization, *Obesity: Preventing and Managing the Global Epidemic*, Who Technical Report Series 894 (Geneva: World Health Organization, 2000).
49 The discourse has shifted slightly from disgust to pity, perhaps as a result of pressure from fat activists, but this is hardly worth celebrating. George Monbiot, "Obesity Is an Incurable Disease. So Why Is the Government Intent on Punishing Sufferers?" *The Guardian*, http://www.theguardian.com/commentisfree/2015/aug/11/obesity-incurable-disease-cameron-punishing-sufferers.

or working at a volunteer fat queer brothel? Through a conviction that something must be done about the problem of fat people or through getting tattooed with a Screaming C? Through a pernicious fantasy of slenderness or through a wink or a rebellious thought? Through all of this or none of it? Queer, fat feminist activism is at the heart of these questions, this radical social movement is the place where answers can be found. Let's look for them together.

BIBLIOGRAPHY

Afful, Adwoa A. and Rose Ricciardelli. "Shaping the Online Fat Acceptance Movement: Talking About Body Image and Beauty Standards." *Journal of Gender Studies* 24, no. 3 (2015): 1-20.

Agel, Joseph. *The Radical Therapist.* New York: Ballantine Books, 1971.

Agger, Ben. "Does Postmodernism Make You Mad? Or, Did You Flunk Statistics?" In *The Sage Handbook of Social Science Methodology*, edited by William Outhwaite and Stephen P. Turner, 443-56. Thousand Oaks, CA: SAGE, 2007.

Ahmed, Sara. *The Promise of Happiness.* Durham, NC: Duke University Press, 2010.

——— "You Are Oppressing Us!" http://feministkilljoys.com/2015/02/15/you-are-oppressing-us/.

Airborne, Max. "True Tales from Life in the Fat Lane." *FaT GiRL* 3 (1995): 48.

Airborne, Max and Cherry Midnight. *Size Queen.* Oakland, CA: Size Queen, 2005.

Aldebaran. "1974 Letter from Aldebaran to Karen Jones." In *The Fat Underground: The Original Radical Fat Feminists - a Commemorative Sourcebook from the Archives of Largesse, the Network for Size Esteem*, edited by Karen Stimson, 56-61. New Haven, CT: Largesse, 1995.

——— "Fat Liberation." *Issues in Radical Therapy* 3, no. Summer (1973).

——— *Health of Fat People: The Scare Story Your Doctor Won't Tell You*. Los Angeles/New Haven, CT: The Fat Underground/Largesse Fat Liberation Archives, 1974. pamphlet.

——— "Letter: Liberal on Fat." *Off Our Backs* 10, no. 3 (1980): 31.

——— "Letter: Oob Perpetuating Stereotypes." *Off Our Backs* 9, no. 11 (1979): 31.

——— "We Are Not Our Enemies." *Sister* December (1973): 6.

Aldebaran, Gudrun, Fonfa, Reanne with Simone, Wallace, Merry, Demarest and Syd Jasso. *A Fat Women's Problem-Solving Group: Radical Change*. Los Angeles/New Haven, CT: The Fat Underground/Largesse Fat Liberation Archives, n.d.

Aldebaran (Vivian Mayer). "Letter: Compulsive Eating Myth." *Off Our Backs* 9, no. 7 (1979): 28.

Alinsky, Saul D. *Rules for Radicals. A Practical Primer from Realistic Radicals*. New York: Vintage Books, 1972.

Allegro Fortissimo. "Allegro Fortissimo." http://www.allegrofortissimo.com/.

Allen, Jamie. "Discussions before an Encounter." *continent* 2, no. 2 (2012): 136-47.

Allied Media Conference. *Research Justice for Movements and Community Voices*. Allied Media Conference. Edited by Allied Media Projects Detroit 2012.

Allison, Michelle. "The Fat Nutritionist." http://www.fatnutritionist.com/.

Andrews-Hunt, Cookie. *Images of Our Flesh*. Seattle: The Fat Avengers, 1983.

Anonymous. "China Daily: 'Fat and Cool' Dance Group Performs." SINA Corporation, http://www.chinadaily.com.cn/photo/2007-09/14/content_6108764.htm.

——— "Curves Have Their Day in Park; 500 at a 'Fat-in' Call for Obesity." *New York Times*, 5 June 1967.

——— "Dimensions." http://www.dimensionsmagazine.com/.

——— "Fat Kids United." https://fatkidsunited.wordpress.com/.

——— "Food for Thought." *Sports Illustrated*, 19 June 1967, 12.

——— *Hunger Strike [Zine]*. In the Spirit of Emma. London. n.d. zine.

——— "National Fat Women's Conference." *Spare Rib*, no. 197 (1988): 89.

——— "Notyourgoodfatty.Com." http://notyourgoodfatty.com/.

——— "Queers Read This." http://www.qrd.org/qrd/misc/text/queers.read.this.

——— "Rachael Field's Paintings." *Spare Rib*, no. 234 (1992): 21.

——— "Rethinking 1000 Fat Cranes." http://blog.twowholecakes. com/2008/09/rethinking-1000-fat-cranes/.

Aphramor, Lucy. "Disability and the Anti-Obesity Offensive." *Disability & Society* 24, no. 7 (2009): 897-909.

——— "Validity of Claims Made in Weight Management Research: A Narrative Review of Dietetic Articles." *Nutrition Journal* 9, no. 30 (2010). http://www.nutritionj.com/content/9/1/30.

Aphramor, Lucy, Yuka Asada, Jennifer Atkins, Shawna Berenbaum, Jenna Brady, Shauna Clarke, John Coveney. "Critical Dietetics: A Declaration." *Practice*, no. 48 (2009): 2.

Armstrong, Elizabeth A. and Mary Bernstein. "Culture, Power, and Institutions: A Multi-Institutional Politics Approach to Social Movements." *Sociological Theory* 26, no. 1 (2008): 74-99.

Asbill, D. Lacy. "'I'm Allowed to Be a Sexual Being': The Distinctive Social Conditions of the Fat Burlesque Stage." In *The Fat Studies Reader*, edited by Esther Rothblum and Sondra Solovay, 299-304. New York: New York University Press, 2009.

Assil Reem, Miho Kim and Saba Waheed. "An Introduction to Research Justice." DataCenter, https://www.z2systems.com/np/clients/datacenter/product. jsp;jsessionid=2F1EEE41401FBEAD18A848DED1D302E7?product=5.

Association for Size Diversity and Health. *Susie Orbach*. Asdah National Conference. Marriott, Dulles VA. 2009.

Atkins, Dawn, ed. *Looking Queer: Body Image and Identity in Lesbian, Bisexual, Gay, and Transgender Communities*. Binghampton, NY: The Haworth Press, 1998.

Atkinson, Paul, Amanda Coffey and Sara Delamont. *Key Themes in Qualitative Research: Continuities and Change*. Walnut Creek, CA: Altamira Press, 2003.

Auerbach, Sara and Rebekah Bradley. "Resistance and Reinscription: Sexual Identity and Body Image among Lesbian and Bisexual Women." In *Looking Queer: Body Image and Identity in Lesbian, Bisexual, Gay, and Transgender Communities*, edited by Dawn Atkins, 27-36. Philadelphia, PA: Haworth Press, 1998.

Avicolli Mecca, Tommi. *Smash the Church, Smash the State! The Early Years of Gay Liberation*. San Francisco: City Lights Books, 2008.

Bacon, Linda, Judith S. Stern, M. D. Van Loan and Nancy L. Keim. "Size Acceptance and Intuitive Eating Improve Health for Obese, Female Chronic Dieters." *Journal of the American Dietetic Association* 105, no. 6 (2005): 929-36.

Bacon, Linda. *Health at Every Size: The Surprising Truth About Your Weight*. Dallas TX: BenBella Books, 2008.

Bacon, Linda and Lucy Aphramor. "Weight Science: Evaluating the Evidence for a Paradigm Shift." *Nutrition Journal* 10, no. 9 (2011). http://www.nutritionj.com/content/10/1/9.

Baker, Jes. *Things No One Will Tell Fat Girls: A Handbook for Unapologetic Living*. Berkeley, CA: Seal Press, 2015.

Baker, Leslie. "Meridith and Judith." *Common Lives/Lesbian Lives* 12 (1984): 27.

Bakhtin, Mikhail. *Rabelais and His World*. Bloomington, IN: Indiana University Press, 1984.

Balkhi, Amanda Marie, Mike C. Parent and Mark Mayor. "Impact of Perceived Weight Discrimination on Patient Satisfaction and Physician Trust." *Fat Studies: An Interdisciplinary Journal of Body Weight and Society* 2, no. 1 (2013): 45-55.

Barbara, Vicki, Marian, Wolfie and Val. "Fat Girl Roundtable 3: Racism and Fat Hatred." *FaT GiRL* 3 (1995): 42-47.

Barron, Kathy, Anne S. Kaplan, Corinna Makris, Lesleigh J. Owen and Frannie Zellman. *Fat Poets Speak: Voices of the Fat Poets Society*. Edited by Frannie Zellman Nashville TN: Pearlsong Press, 2009.

Barron, Nancy. "I Like the Me I'm Becoming." In *Journeys to Self-Acceptance: Fat Women Speak*, edited by Carol Wiley, 112-23. Freedom, CA: The Crossing Press, 1994.

Barron, Nancy and B.H. Lear. "Ample Opportunity for Fat Women." *Women and Therapy* 8 (1989): 79-82.

Barron, Nancy, Lucia Eakins and Richard Wollert. "Fat Group: A Snap-Launched Self-Help Group for Overweight Women." *Human Organization* 43, no. 1 (1984): 44-49.

Bartky, Sandra Lee. "Foucault, Femininity and the Modernisation of Patriarchal Power." In *Feminism and Foucault: Paths of Resistance*, edited by Lee Quinby and Irene Diamond, 61-86. Boston: Northeastern University Press, 1988.

Bas Hannah, Sharon. "Naomi Cohen Choked on the Culture." *Sister* September (1974): 1.

Basham, Patrick, Gio B. Gori and John Luik. *Diet Nation: Exposing the Obesity Crusade*. London: Social Affairs Unit. 2006.

Bass, Margaret K. "On Being a Fat Black Girl in a Fat-Hating Culture." In *Recovering the Black Female Body: Self-Representations by African American Women*, edited by Michael Bennett and Vanessa D. Dickerson, 219-30. New Brunswick, NJ: Rutgers University Press, 2001.

Baumgardner, Jennifer and Amy Richards. *Manifesta: Young Women, Feminism and the Future*. New York: Farrar, Straus and Giroux, 2000.

BBC. *Fat Women Here to Stay, Open Space*. UK, 1989. Television.

——— *Fat Women Here to Stay*. Open Space. Edited by Community Programme Unit. UK. 1989. Television.

——— *Wogan*. UK. 1989. Television.

Bean, Linda, Beverley Duguid and Barbara Burford. "Body Consciousness." *Spare Rib* 182 (1987): 20-21.

Beckett, Angharad E. "Understanding Social Movements: Theorising the Disability Movement in Conditions of Late Modernity." *The Sociological Review* 54, no. 4 (2006): 734-52.

Bell, Susan E. "Sexualizing Research: Response to Erich Goode." *Qualitative Sociology* 25, no. 4 (2002): 535-39.

Berlant, Lauren. "Slow Death (Sovereignty, Obesity, Lateral Agency)." *Critical Inquiry* 33 (2007): 754-80.

Big Liberty. "The Fat Liberation Feed." http://biglibertyblog.com/the-fat-liberation-feed/.

Black, Carol. "An Independent Review into the Impact on Employment Outcomes of Drug or Alcohol Addiction, and Obesity." Edited by Department for Work and Pensions. London: Government of the United

Kingdon, 2015.

Blank, Hanne. *Big Big Love: A Sourcebook on Sex for People of Size.* Emeryville, CA: The Greenery Press, 2000.

——— *Zaftig! Sex for the Well Rounded [Zine].* Boston MA: Zaftig! Productions. 1999.

Bobel, Chris. "'I'm Not an Activist Though I've Done a Lot of It': Doing Activism, Being Activist and the 'Perfect Standard' in a Contemporary Movement." *Social Movement Studies* 6, no. 2 (2007): 147-59.

Boero, Natalie. *Killer Fat.* New Brunswick, NJ: Rutgers University Press, 2012.

Bombaka, Andrea E. "'Obesities': Experiences and Perspectives across Weight Trajectories." *Health Sociology Review* (2015): 1-14.

Bordo, Susan. "Feminism, Foucault and the Politics of the Body." In *Feminist Theory and the Body: A Reader*, edited by Janet Price and Margrit Shildrick, 246-57. Edinburgh: Edinburgh University Press, 1999.

——— *Unbearable Weight: Feminism, Western Culture, and the Body.* 10th anniversary ed. Berkeley, CA: University of California Press, 2003.

Bosky, Bernadette Lynn. "Some Painful and Healing Words." In *Journeys to Self-Acceptance: Fat Women Speak*, edited by Carol Wiley, 54-64. Freedom, CA: The Crossing Press, 1994.

Boston Womens Health Collective. *The New Our Bodies, Ourselves.* New York: Simon & Schuster, 1984.

Bourdieu, Pierre and Loïc Wacquant. "Language, Gender and Symbolic Violence." In *An Invitation to Reflexive Sociology.* Edited by Pierre Bourdieu and Loïc Wacquant, 140-74. Cambridge: Polity, 1992.

Bourdieu, Pierre. "The Forms of Capital." In *Handbook of Theory and Research for the Sociology of Education*. Edited by John G. Richardson. 241-58. New York: Greenwood, 1986.

Bourdieu, Pierre. *Distinction: A Social Critique of the Judgement of Taste*. Cambridge, MA: Harvard University Press, 1984.

Bovey, Shelley. *Being Fat Is Not a Sin*. London: Pandora, 1989.

——— *What Have You Got to Lose? The Great Weight Debate and How to Diet Successfully*. London: The Women's Press, 2001.

——— *The Forbidden Body: Why Being Fat Is Not a Sin*. London: Pandora, 1994.

——— *Sizeable Reflections: Big Women Living Full Lives*. London: Women's Press, 2000.

Bradya, Jennifer, Jacqui Gingras and Lucy Aphramor. "Theorizing Health at Every Size as a Relational–Cultural Endeavour." *Critical Public Health* 23, no. 3 (2013): 345–55.

Brandheim, Susanne. "The Misrecognition Mind-Set: A Trap in the Transformative Responsibility of Critical Weight Studies." *Distinktion: Scandinavian Journal of Social Theory* 13, no. 1 (2012): 93-108.

Brandon, Toby and Gary Pritchard. "'Being Fat': A Conceptual Analysis Using Three Models of Disability." *Disability & Society* 26, no. 1 (2011): 79-82.

Branlandingham, Bevin. "The Queer Fat Femme Guide to Life." http://queerfatfemme.com/.

Braziel, Jana Evans and Kathleen LeBesco. *Bodies out of Bounds: Fatness and Transgression*. Berkeley: University of California Press, 2001.

Brittingham, Kimberly. "Fat Is Contagious." http://www.freshyarn. com/42/essays/brittingham_fat1.htm.

Brittingham, Kim. *Read My Hips: How I Learned to Love My Body, Ditch Dieting and Live Large*. New York: Random House, 2011.

Bronstein, Carolyn. "Fat Acceptance Blogging, Female Bodies and the Politics of Emotion." *Feral Feminisms*, no. 3 (2015): 106-18.

Brooks, L. "Size Matters." http://www.shelleybovey.com/frameset.html?/ sizematters.html.

Brown, Laurence. "Fat Is a Bearish Issue." In *The Bear Book II: Further Readings in the History and Evolution of a Gay Male Subculture*. Edited by Les K. Wright. 39-54. New York: Haworth Press, 2001.

Brown, Sonya. "An Obscure Middle Ground: Size Acceptance Narratives and Photographs of 'Real Women.'" *Feminist Media Studies* 5, no. 2 (2005): 237-60.

Brownell, Kelly D., Leslie Rudd, Marlene B. Schwartz and Rebecca M. Puhl. *Weight Bias: Nature, Consequences, and Remedies*. New York: Guildford Press, 2005.

Bruno Altman, Barbara. "The Haes® Files: History of the Health at Every Size® Movement." Association for Size Diversity and Health. http://healthateverysizeblog.org/2013/04/30/ the-haes-files-history-of-the-health-at-every-size-movement-part-i/.

Burford, Barbara. "The Landscapes Painted on the inside of My Skin." *Spare Rib*, no. 179 (1987): 36-39.

Burford, James and Sam Orchard. "Chubby Boys with Strap-Ons: Queering Fat Transmasculine Embodiment." In *Queering Fat Embodiment*. Edited by Cat Pausé, Jackie Wykes and Samantha Murray. 61-74. Farnham: Ashgate, 2014.

Butland, Bryony, Susan Jebb, Peter Kopelman, Klim McPherson, Sandy Thomas, Jane Mardell and Vivienne Parry. *Foresight Tackling Obesities: Future Choices – Project Report*. London: Government Office for Science, 2005.

Butler, Judith. *Undoing Gender*. New York: Routledge, 2004.

——— *Precarious Life: The Powers of Mourning and Violence*. London: Verso, 2004.

——— *Gender Trouble: Feminism and the Subversion of Identity*. New York: Routledge, 2006.

Cade, Cathy. *A Lesbian Photo Album: The Lives of Seven Lesbian Feminists*. Oakland, CA: Waterwoman Books, 1987.

Cahill, Ann J. "Getting to My Fighting Weight." *Hypatia* 25, no. 2 (2010): 485-92.

Califia, Patrick. *Public Sex: The Culture of Radical Sex*. 2nd ed. San Francisco: Cleis Press, 2000.

Cameron, Erin. "Teaching Resources for Post-Secondary Educators Who Challenge Dominant 'Obesity' Discourse." *Fat Studies: An Interdisciplinary Journal of Body Weight and Society* 4, no. 2 (2015).

Campbell, Drew. "Confessions of a Fat Sex Worker." In *Whores and Other Feminists*. Edited by Jill Nagle. 189-90. New York: Routledge, 1997.

Campos, Paul F. *The Diet Myth: Why America's Obsession with Weight Is Hazardous to Your Health*. New York: Gotham Books, 2005.

Campos, Paul F., Abigail Saguy, Paul Ernsberger, Eric Oliver and Glenn Gaesser. "The Epidemiology of Overweight and Obesity: Public Health Crisis or Moral Panic?" *International Journal of Epidemiology* 35, no. 1 (2006): 55-60.

Campos, Paul F. *The Obesity Myth: Why America's Obsession with Weight Is Hazardous to Your Health*. New York: Gotham Books, 2004.

Cantrell, Amber. "Freaking Fatness through History: Critical Intersections of Fatness and Disability." *Chrestomathy: Annual Review of Undergraduate Research* 12 (2013): 1-39.

Cartwright, Richard L. "Some Remarks on Essentialism." *The Journal of Philosophy* 65, no. 20 (1968): 615-26.

Casio, Holly. "Joining the Dots: A Queer Fat Positive Perzine About Pcos." 2012.

Cathy and Zhana. "Fat Women Celebrate!" *Spare Rib* no. 216 (1990): 55.

Cattell, Maria G. and Jacob G. Climo. "Introduction: Meaning in Social Memory and History: Anthropological Perspectives." In *Social Memory and History: Anthropological Perspectives*. Edited by Jacob G. Climo and Maria G. Cattell. 1-38. Walnut Creek, CA: AltaMira Press, 2002.

Chalklin, Vikki. "All Hail the Fierce Fat Femmes." In *Fat Sex: New Directions in Theory and Activism*. Edited by Helen Hester and Caroline Walters. 104-19. Farnham: Ashgate, 2014.

Chang, Heewon. *Autoethnography as Method*. Walnut Creek, CA: Left Coast Press, 2008.

Chapkis, Wendy. *Beauty Secrets: Women and the Politics of Appearance*. London: The Women's Press, 1986.

Chastain, Ragen. *Fat: The Owner's Manual: Navigating a Thin-Obsessed World with Your Health, Happiness, and Self-Esteem Intact*. Austin, TX: Sized for Success Multimedia, LLC, 2012.

Cheek, Julianne. "Healthism: A New Conservatism?" *Qualitative Health Research* 18, no. 7 (2008): 974-82.

Chernin, Kim. *The Hungry Self: Women, Eating and Identity*. New York: Times Books, 1985.

———— *The Obsession: Reflections on the Tyranny of Slenderness*. New York: Harper & Row, 1981.

———— *Womansize: The Tyranny of Slenderness*. London: The Women's Press, 1983.

Christine and Deva. *Heavy SM: Fat Brats Speak Out*. Edited by Fish San Francisco: Brat Attack: The Zine for Leatherdykes and Other Bad Girls [zine]. 1991.

Clarke, Danielle. "Finding the Subject: Queering the Archive." *Feminist Theory* 5, no. 1 (2004): 79-83.

Cochrane, Kira. "The Reluctant Dieter." *The Guardian*. http://www.theguardian.com/lifeandstyle/series/thereluctantdieter.

———— "Young, Fat and Fabulous." *The Guardian*. http://www.guardian.co.uk/theguardian/2010/jan/30/fat-fashion-blogs.

Coffey, Amanda. *The Ethnographic Self: Fieldwork and the Representation of Identity*. London: SAGE, 1999.

Colls, Rachel. "Big Girls Having Fun: Reflections on a 'Fat Accepting Space.'" *Somatechnics* 2, no. 1 (2012): 18-37.

Colls, Rachel and Bethan Evans. "Making Space for Fat Bodies? A Critical Account of 'the Obesogenic Environment.'" *Progress in Human Geography* 1, no. 21 (2013).

Cooper, Charlotte. "Charlotte Cooper and Judy Freespirit in Conversation, June 2010." http://obesitytimebomb.blogspot.com/2010/09/charlotte-cooper-and-judy-freespirit-in.html.

——— "Olympics/Uhlympics: Living in the Shadow of the Beast." *thirdspace* 9, no. 2 (2010).

——— "Can a Fat Woman Call Herself Disabled?" *Disability & Society* 12, no. 1 (February 1997): 31-41.

——— "The Chubsters." http://charlottecooper.net/b/chubsters/.

——— "Fat Activism in Ten Astonishing, Beguiling, Inspiring and Beautiful Episodes." In *Fat Studies in the Uk*. Edited by Corinna Tomrley and Ann Kaloski Naylor. 19-31. York: Raw Nerve Books, 2009.

——— "Fat Studies: Mapping the Field." *Sociology Compass* 4, no. 12 (2010): 1020-34.

——— "Fattylympics." http://fattylympics.blogspot.co.uk/.

——— "Headless Fatties, the Visual Cliché That Will Not Die." http://obesitytimebomb.blogspot.co.uk/2012/01/headless-fatties-visual-cliche-that.html.

——— "Hey Sisters, Welcome to My World." In *Hot&Heavy: Fierce Fat Girls on Life, Love and Fashion*. Edited by Virgie Tovar. 65-70. Berkeley,

CA: Seal Press, 2012.

——— "I Am a Fat Dancer, but I Am Not Your Inspiration Porn." *OpenDemocracy*. https://www.opendemocracy.net/transformation/charlotte-cooper/i-am-fat-dancer-but-i-am-not-your-inspiration-porn.

——— "No More Stitch-Ups: Media Literacy for Fat Activists." http://obesitytimebomb.blogspot.co.uk/2013/05/no-more-stitch-ups-media-literacy-for.html.

——— "Political and Social Group for Other Fat Women." *Spare Rib*, no. 233 (1992): 48.

——— "A Queer and Trans Fat Activist Timeline - Zine Download." http://charlottecooper.net/b/oral-history/a-queer-and-trans-fat-activist-timeline/.

——— "A Queer and Trans Fat Activist Timeline: Queering Fat Activist Nationality and Cultural Imperialism." *Fat Studies: An Interdisciplinary Journal of Body Weight and Society* 1, no. 1 (2012): 61-74.

——— "Rad Fatty: Corinna Tomrley." http://www.obesitytimebomb.blogspot.co.uk/2009/07/rad-fatty-corinna-tomrley.html.

——— "The Story of the Chubsters." In *Pop Culture Association/American Culture Association*. Edited by L. Owen and J. McCrossin. Marriott, New Orleans, 2009.

——— "Chubsters Vs Imps." *Cheap Date*, 2005, 16-20.

——— *Fat & Proud: The Politics of Size*. London: The Women's Press, 1998.

——— "How to Ride a Bike: A Guide for Fat Cyclists." http://

charlottecooper.net/publishing/digital/how-to-ride-a-bike-a-guide-for-fat-cyclists-02-05/.

———— "The Six Types of Obesity Researcher." Obesity Timebomb. http://obesitytimebomb.blogspot.co.uk/2015/04/the-six-types-of-obesity-researcher.html.

Cooper, Charlotte and Kay Hyatt. "Big Bum Jumble." http://www.bigbumjumble.blogspot.co.uk/.

Cooper, Charlotte and Samantha Murray. "Fat Activist Community: A Conversation Piece." *Somatechnics* 2, no. 1 (2012): 127-38.

Cooper, Charlotte, Rachel White, Kay Hyatt and Simon Murphy. "Big Bums [Zine]." London, 2008.

Courtney, Jeanne. "Size Acceptance as a Grief Process: Observations from Psychotherapy with Lesbian Feminists." *Journal of Lesbian Studies* 12, no. 4 (2008): 347-63.

Crenshaw, Kimberlé. "Demarginalizing the Intersection of Race and Sex: A Black Feminist Critique of Antidiscrimination Doctrine, Feminist Theory and Antiracist Politics." *University of Chicago Legal Forum* (1989): 139-67.

Crossley, Nick. "Fat Is a Sociological Issue: Obesity Rates in Late Modern, 'Body-Conscious' Societies." *Social Theory & Health* 2 (2004): 222-53.

———— "Sociology and the Body." In *The Sage Handbook of Sociology*. Edited by Craig Calhoun, Chris Rojek and Bryan Turner. London: SAGE, 2005.

CSWD. "Council on Size and Weight Discrimination." http://www.cswd.org/.

Curtis, Ted, Robert Dellar, Esther Leslie and Ben Watson. *Mad Pride: A Celebration of Mad Culture.* London: Spare Change Books, 2000.

Cusitar, Leanne, Sherece Taffe, Mariko Tamaki, Allyson Mitchell, Abi Sloane, Kerry Daniels-Zraidi and T.J. Bryan, eds. *The Fat Issue.* Edited by Caroline Sin, Shauna Lancit and Jessica Ticktin. Vol. 67, *Fireweed.* Toronto, Ontario: Fireweed, 1999.

Cvetkovich, Ann. *An Archive of Feelings: Trauma, Sexuality, and Lesbian Public Cultures.* Durham, NC: Duke University Press, 2003.

D., Katie. "Rolls with Butter: A Fat Activist Zine." n.d.

Dailey, Kate. "'Fatshion' Blogs Defiantly Celebrate Plus-Size Couture." *BBC.* http://www.bbc.co.uk/news/magazine-16259070.

Daníelsdóttir, Sigrún, Deb Burgard, and Wendy Oliver-Pyatt. "Academy for Eating Disorders Guidelines for Childhood Obesity Prevention Programs." Academy for Eating Disorders. http://aedweb.org/web/index.php/23-get-involved/position-statements/90-aed-statement-on-body-shaming-and-weight-prejudice-in-public-endeavors-to-reduce-obesity-4.

DataCenter. "Research Justice." http://www.datacenter.org/research-justice/.

Davis, Angela Y. *Are Prisons Obsolete?* New York: Seven Stories Press, 2003.

Davis, Kathy. *The Making of Our Bodies, Ourselves: How Feminism Travels across Borders.* Durham, NC and London: Duke University Press, 2007.

Debord, Guy. *The Society of the Spectacle.* St Petersburg FL: Black & Red, 1984.

Della Porta, Donatella and Mario Diani. *Social Movements: An Introduction*. Second edition. Oxford: Blackwell, 2006.

Deller, Robert. *Splitting in Two: Mad Pride and Punk Rock Oblivion*. London: Unkant Publishers, 2014.

Diamond, Nicky. "Thin Is the Feminist Issue." *Feminist Review* 19 (1985): 45-64.

Dickins, Marissa, Samantha L. Thomas, Bri King, Sophie Lewis and Kate Holland. "The Role of the Fatosphere in Fat Adults' Responses to Obesity Stigma: A Model of Empowerment without a Focus on Weight Loss." *Qualitative Health Research* 21, no. 12 (2011): 1679-91.

Ditto, Beth and Michelle Tea. *Coal to Diamonds*. London: Simon & Schuster, 2012.

Donaghue, Ngaire. "The Moderating Effects of Socioeconomic Status on Relationships between Obesity Framing and Stigmatization of Fat People." *Fat Studies: An Interdisciplinary Journal of Body Weight and Society* 3, no. 1 (2014): 6-16.

Donald, Christine M. *The Fat Woman Measures Up*. Charlottetown, P.E.I: Ragweed, 1986.

Downes, Julia, Maddie Breeze and Naomi Griffin. "Researching DIY Cultures: Towards a Situated Ethical Practice for Activist-Academia." *Graduate Journal of Social Science* 10, no. 3 (2013).

Downing Peters, Lauren. "Queering the Hourglass: Beauty and New Wave Fat Activism." In *Beauty: Exploring Critical Issues*. Oxford, UK, 2013.

Drinkwater, Kelli Jean. "Aquaporko: The Documentary." http://aquaporkofilm.com/.

DuBois, James M., Ana S. Ilitis and Susan G. DuBois, eds. *Narrative Inquiry in Bioethics.* Volume 4. Number 2. Baltimore, MD: The Johns Hopkins University Press, 2014.

Dudley, Betty Rose. "A Fat, Vulgar, Angry, Slut." *FaT GiRL* 4 (1995): 21-22.

Duggan, Lisa. *The Twilight of Equality: Neoliberalism, Cultural Politics and the Attack on Democracy.* Boston: Beacon Press, 2003.

Dunham, Kelli. "I Promise You Can Successfully Get a Pap Exam Even If You Are Traumatized, Grossed out or Really Really Not into Those Parts." xojane. http://www.xojane.com/healthy/i-promise-you-can-get-a-pap-exam-even-if-you-are-traumatized-weirded-out-grossed-out-or-really-really-not-into-those-bits.

Durden, Krissy. *Figure 8 [Zine].* Portland, OR: Ponyboy Press. 2001-2009.

Dykewomon, Elana. "Changing the World." In *Everyday Mutinies: Funding Lesbian Activism.* Edited by Nanette Gartrell and Esther D. Rothblum. 53-62. Binghampton: Harrington Park Press, 2001.

——— "Fat Liberation." In *Encyclopedia of Lesbian and Gay Histories and Cultures, Volume 1.* Edited by George Haggerty and Bonnie Zimmerman. 290-91. New York: Garland, 2000.

——— "Lesbian Quarters." *Journal of Lesbian Studies* 9, no. 1-2 (2005): 31-43.

——— "Travelling Fat." In *Shadow on a Tightrope: Writings by Women on Fat Oppression.* Edited by Lisa Schoenfielder and Barb Wieser. 144-54. Iowa City: Aunt Lute, 1983.

Dyson, Sue. *A Weight Off Your Mind: How to Stop Worrying About Your Body Size.* London: Sheldon Press, 1991.

Earl, Jennifer. "Political Repression: Iron Fists, Velvet Gloves, and Diffuse Control." *Annual Review of Sociology* 37, no. 1 (2011): 261-84.

Earthdaughter, debby. "Letter: Diet Pills Next?" *Off Our Backs* 21, no. 3 (1991): 35.

Edison, Laurie Toby and Debbie Notkin. *Women En Large: Images of Fat Nudes.* 1st ed. San Francisco, CA: Books in Focus, 1994.

Edwards, Elizabeth A. "Letter: Weight Oppression." *Off Our Backs* 19, no. 8 (1989): 26.

Edwards, Tim. "Queer Fears: Against the Cultural Turn." *Sexualities* 1, no. 4 (1998): 471-84.

Ehrenreich, Barbara. *Smile or Die: How Positive Thinking Fooled America and the World.* London: Granta, 2010.

Elg, Theresa. "Letter: Weight Ad Unacceptable." *Off Our Backs* 21, no. 5 (1991): 34.

Ellis, Carolyn. *The Ethnographic I: A Methodological Novel About Autoethnography.* Walnut Creek, CA: AltaMira Press, 2004.

Ellison, Jenny. "Weighing In: The 'Evidence of Experience' and Canadian Fat Women's Activism." *Canadian Bulletin of Medical History / Bulletin canadien d'histoire de la médicine* 30, no. 1 (2013): 55-75.

Eng, David L., Judith Halberstam and José Esteban Muñoz. "What's Queer About Queer Studies Now?" *Social Text* 23, no. 3-4 (2005): 1-17.

Erdman Farrell, Amy. *Fat Shame: Stigma and the Fat Body in American Culture.* New York: New York University Press, 2011.

Evans, Bethan and Rachel Colls. "Measuring Fatness, Governing Bodies: The Spatialities of the Body Mass Index (Bmi) in Anti-Obesity Politics." *Antipode: A Radical Journal of Geography* 41, no. 5 (2009): 1051-83.

Evans, John, Emma Rich, Brian Davies, Rachel Allwood. *Education, Disordered Eating and Obesity Discourse: Fat Fabrications.* Abingdon: Routledge, 2008.

Evans Young, Mary. *Diet Breaking: Having It All without Having to Diet.* London: Hodder & Stoughton, 1995.

Fabrey, W. J. "Thirty-Three Years of Size Acceptance in Perspective- How Has It Affected the Lives of Real People?" http://members.tripod. com/~bigastexas/2001event/keynote2001.html

Fabrey, W. J. Email, 10 August 2008.

Fabrey, W.J. Email, 4 January 2009.

Faircloth, Kelly. "Fatshion Police: How Plus-Size Blogging Left Its Radical Roots Behind." *The New York Observer.* http://betabeat.com/2013/02/ fatshion-plus-size-bloggers-amanda-piasecki-marianne-kirby-gabrielle-gregg/.

FaT GiRL Collective. *Fat Girl.* San Francisco, CA: FaT GiRL, 1994.

Fat Lip Reader's Theatre. *Nothing to Lose [Video].* Oakland, CA: Wolfe Video, 1989. Video.

Fat Women's Group. "Fat Women's Group." *Spare Rib,* no. 208 (1989): 88.

Fiegel, Eddi. *Dream a Little Dream of Me: The Life of 'Mama' Cass Elliot.* London: Pan, 2006.

Fife, Kirsty. "Hard Femme." 2013-2015.

——— "I Love Myself: A Self Care Zine." n.d.

——— "Make It Work #2." n.d.

——— "Make It Work: A Diy Fatshion Zine." Leeds, 2012.

Fink, Marty. "It Gets Fatter: Graphic Fatness and Resilient Eating in Mariko and Jillian Tamaki's Skim." *Fat Studies: An Interdisciplinary Journal of Body Weight and Society* 2, no. 2 (2013): 132-46.

Fishman, Sara Golda Bracha. "Life in the Fat Underground." http://www.radiancemagazine.com/issues/1998/winter_98/fat_underground.html.

Flores, April. "Voluptuous Life." In *Hot & Heavy: Fierce Fat Girls on Life, Lover & Fashion*. Edited by Virgie Tovar. 121-25. Berkeley, CA: Seal Press, 2012.

Foster, Jill. "The Roly-Poly Olympics!" Associated Newspapers. http://www.dailymail.co.uk/news/article-2170666/Fattylympics-The-Roly-poly-Olympics-Contestants-WERE-game-laugh.html#ixzz20DL84C4t.

Foucault, Michel and Colin Gordon. *Power/Knowledge: Selected Interviews and Other Writings, 1972-1977*. Brighton: The Harvester Press, 1980.

Foucault, Michel. *Discipline and Punish: The Birth of the Prison*. New York: Random House, 1977.

——— *The History of Sexuality, Vol. 1*. Harmondsworth: Penguin, 1981.

——— "Power and Strategies." In *Power/Knowledge: Selected Interviews and Other Writings, 1972-1977*. Edited by Michel Foucault and Colin Gordon. 134-45. Brighton: The Harvester Press, 1980.

———— "The Subject and Power." In *Michel Foucault: Beyond Structuralism and Hermeneutics*, edited by Hubert Dreyfus and Paul Rabinow. Chicago: University of Chicago Press, 1982.

Foucault, Michel and Jay Miskowiec. "Of Other Spaces." Architecture / Mouvement/ Continuité. http://foucault.info/documents/heteroTopia/ foucault.heteroTopia.en.html.

Fraser, Nancy. "Injustice at Intersecting Scales: On 'Social Exclusion' and the 'Global Poor.'" *European Journal of Social Theory* 13, no. 3 (2010): 363-71.

———— "Rethinking the Public Sphere: A Contribution to the Critique of Actually Existing Democracy." *Social Text* 25, no. 26 (1990): 56-80.

———— "Who Counts? Dilemmas of Justice in a Postwestphalian World." *Antipode* 41 (2009): 281-197.

Frater, Lara. *Fat Chicks Rule! How to Survive in a Thin-Centric World.* New York: Ig Publishing, 2005.

Freeperson, Kathy. "Letter: Heavy Punishment." *Off Our Backs* 13, no. 5 (1983): 30.

Freespirit, Judy and Aldebaran. "Writings from the Fat Underground." In *Shadow on a Tightrope: Writings by Women on Fat Oppression.* Edited by Lisa Schoenfielder and Barb Wieser. 52-57. Iowa City: Aunt Lute, 1983.

Freespirit, Judy. "Doing Donahue." *Common Lives/Lesbian Lives* 20 (1986): 5-14.

———— *A Slim Volume of Fat Poems.* Oakland CA: Judy Freespirit, 1996.

Freespirit, Judy and Aldebaran. *Fat Liberation Manifesto.* Largesse Fat

Liberation Archives. Edited by The Fat Underground Los Angeles/New Haven, CT: The Fat Underground/Largesse Fat Liberation Archives, 1973.

Freire, Paulo. *Pedagogy of the Oppressed.* 2nd Edition. London: Penguin, 1970.

French, Dawn. *Dear Fatty.* London: Century, 2008.

Friedli, Lynne and Robert Stearn. "Positive Affect as Coercive Strategy: Conditionality, Activation and the Role of Psychology in Uk Government Workfare Programmes." *Medical Humanities* 41, no. 1 (2015): 40-47.

Friedman, Abraham I. *Fat Can Be Beautiful: Stop Dieting, Start Living.* Berekeley, CA: Berekeley Publishing Corporation, 1974.

Friedman, Jeffrey M. "A War on Obesity, Not the Obese." *Science* 299, no. 5608 (2003): 856-59.

Friedman, May. "Fat Is a Social Work Issue: Fat Bodies, Moral Regulation, and the History of Social Work." *Intersectionalities: A Global Journal of 2012 Social Work Analysis, Research, Polity, and Practice* 1 (2012): 53-69.

Fumento, Michael. *The Fat of the Land: The Obesity Epidemic and How Overweight Americans Can Help Themselves.* New York: Viking/Allen Lane, 1997.

Gaesser, Glen. *Big Fat Lies: The Truth About Your Weight and Your Health.* Carlsbad, CA: Gurze Books, 2002.

Gailey, Jeannine A. "Fat Shame to Fat Pride: Fat Women's Sexual and Dating Experiences." *Fat Studies: An Interdisciplinary Journal of Body Weight and Society* 1, no. 1 (2012): 114-27.

Ganz, Johnanna J. "'The Bigger, the Better': Challenges in Portraying a Positive Fat Character in Weeds." *Fat Studies: An Interdisciplinary Journal of Body Weight and Society* 1, no. 2 (2012): 208-21.

Gard, Lauren. "Fat-Is-Beautiful Activist Marilyn Wann Protests Japan's Thinness Law." *SF Weekly*. http://www.sfweekly.com/2008-08-27/news/fat-is-beautiful-activist-marilyn-wann-protests-japan-s-thinness-law/.

Gard, Michael. *The End of the Obesity Epidemic*. Abingdon: Routledge, 2011.

Gard, Michael and Jan Wright. *The Obesity Epidemic: Science, Morality, and Ideology*. Abingdon: Routledge, 2005.

Gay & Lesbian Arts and Media. "Before Stonewall: A Lesbian, Gay, Bisexual and Transgendered Oral History." London, 2004.

Gerber, Lynne. "Movements of Luxurious Exuberence: Georges Bataille and Fat Politics." In *Negative Ecstasies: Georges Bataille and the Study of Religion*. Edited by Jeremy Biles and Kent L. Brintnall. 19-37. New York: Fordham University Press, 2015.

Gibbons, Brittany. *Fat Girl Walking: Sex, Food, Love, and Being Comfortable in Your Skin...Every Inch of It*. New York: Dey Street Books/HarperCollins, 2015.

Giffney, Noreen. "Introduction: The 'Q' Word." In *The Ashgate Research Companion to Queer Theory*. Edited by Noreen Giffney and Michael O'Rourke. 1-13. Farnham: Ashgate, 2009.

Giffney, Noreen and Michael O'Rourke. *The Ashgate Research Companion to Queer Theory*. Farnham: Ashgate, 2009.

Gilman, Sander. *Fat: A Cultural History of Obesity*. Boston: Polity, 2008.

Gimlin, Debra L. *Body Work: Beauty and Self-Image in American Culture*.

Berkeley: University of California Press, 2002.

Gingras, Jacqueline Rochelle. *Longing for Recognition: The Joys, Complexities, and Contradictions of Practicing Dietetics*. York: Raw Nerve, 2009.

Gingras, Jacqui and Charlotte Cooper. "Down the Rabbit Hole: A Critique of the * in Haes®." *Journal of Critical Dietetics* 1, no. 3 (2013): 2-5.

Goffman, Erving. *Stigma: Notes on the Management of Spoiled Identity*. London: Penguin, 1963.

Goode, Erich. "Sexual Involvement and Social Research in a Fat Civil Rights Organization." *Qualitative Sociology* 25, no. 4 (2002): 501-34.

Goode, Erich and J. Preissler. "The Fat Admirer." *Deviant Behavior* 4 (1983): 175-202.

Goodman, W. Charisse. *The Invisible Woman: Confronting Weight Prejudice in America*. Carlsbad CA: Gurze Books, 1995.

Gough, Brendan and Gareth Flanders. "Celebrating 'Obese' Bodies: Gay 'Bears' Talk About Weight, Body Image and Health." *International Journal of Men's Health* 8, no. 3 (2009): 235-53.

Graham-Leigh, Elaine. *A Diet of Austerity: Class, Food and Climate Change*. London: Zero Books, 2015.

Graves, Jennifer L. and Samantha Kwan. "Is There Really 'More to Love'?: Gender, Body, and Relationship Scripts in Romance-Based Reality Television." *Fat Studies: An Interdisciplinary Journal of Body Weight and Society* 1, no. 1 (2012): 47-60.

Grossman, Jennifer. "The Perils of 'Fat Acceptance." *National Review*

55, no. 22 (2003): 34-38.

Grosswirth, Marvin. *Fat Pride: A Survival Handbook.* New York: Jarrow Press, 1971.

Grosz, Elizabeth. *Volatile Bodies: Towards a Corporeal Feminism.* Bloomington, IN: Indiana University Press, 1994.

Gurrieri, Lauren. "Stocky Bodies: Fat Visual Activism." *Fat Studies: An Interdisciplinary Journal of Body Weight and Society* 2, no. 2 (2013): 197-209.

Guthman, Julie. "Teaching the Politics of Obesity: Insights into Neoliberal Embodiment and Contemporary Biopolitics." *Antipode: A Radical Journal of Geography* 41, no. 5 (2009): 1110-1133.

Guthman, Julie and Melanie DuPuis. "Embodying Neoliberalism: Economy, Culture, and the Politics of Fat." *Environment and Planning D: Society and Space* 24 (2006): 427-48.

Habermas, Jürgen. *The Structural Transformation of the Public Sphere: An Inquiry into a Category of Bourgeois Society.* Translated by Thomas Burger and Frederick Lawrence. Cambridge: Polity Press, 1989.

Halberstam, Jack, Gayatri Gopinath, Lisa Duggan, Tavia Nyong'o, Ann Pellegrini and José Muñoz. "Bullybloggers on Failure and the Future of Queer Studies." Bully Bloggers. http://bullybloggers.wordpress.com/2012/04/02/bullybloggers-on-failure-and-the-future-of-queer-studies/.

Halberstam, Judith. "The Anti-Social Turn in Queer Studies." *Graduate Journal of Social Science* 5, no. 2 (2008): 140-56.

——— *In a Queer Time & Place: Transgender Bodies, Subcultural Lives.* New York: New York University Press, 2005.

Hanhardt, Christina B. *The Safe Space: Gay Neighborhood History and the Politics of Violence*. Durham, NC: Duke University Press, 2013.

Harding, Kate. "Dear Naafa." http://kateharding.net/2007/06/24/dear-naafa/.

Harding, Kate and Marianne Kirby. *Lessons from the Fat-O-Sphere: Quit Dieting and Declare a Truce with Your Body*. New York: Perigee, 2009.

Harjunen, Hannele. *Women and Fat: Approaches to the Social Study of Fatness*. Jyväskylä Studies in Education, Psychology and Social Research. Jyväskylä: Jyväskylän Yliopisto, 2010.

Harjunen, Hannele. "Exploring Obesity through the Social Model of Disability." In *Gender and Disability Research in the Nordic Countries*. Edited by Rannveig; Traustadóttir and Kristjana Kristiansen. 305-24. Lund: Studentlitteratur, 2004.

——— "Normality Is Overrated." *NormiHomoLehti*. 2011. 16-19.

Harvey, David. *A Brief History of Neoliberalism*. Oxford: Oxford University Press, 2007.

Hayman, Amanda. "Fat Oppression." *Gossip: A Journal of Lesbian Feminist Ethics* 3 (1986): 66-72.

Heffernan, Karen. "Lesbians and the Internalization of Societal Standards of Weight and Appearance." *Journal of Lesbian Studies* 3, no. 4 (1999): 121-27.

Hernandez, A. "Judy Freespirit." *FaT GiRL* 1 (1994): 6-7.

Herndon, April. "Disparate but Disabled: Fat Embodiment and Disability Studies." *National Women's Studies Association Journal* 14, no. 3 (2002): 121-37.

Hester, Helen and Caroline Walters. *Fat Sex: New Directions in Theory and Activism*. Farnham: Ashgate, 2015.

Hinckley, David. "New York Radio Contrarian and Wnyc Morning Host Steve Post Dies at Age 70." http://www.nydailynews.com/entertainment/new-york-radio-show-host-steve-post-dies-age-70-article-1.1890789.

Hoffman, Abbie. *Revolution for the Hell of It*. New York: Dial Press, 1970.

Hollibaugh, Amber. "Queers without Money: They Are Everywhere. But We Refuse to See Them." http://www.villagevoice.com/2001-06-19/news/queers-without-money/.

hooks, bell. *Outlaw Culture: Resisting Representations*. New York: Routledge, 1994.

——— *Teaching to Transgress: Education as the Practice of Freedom*. New York: Routledge, 1994.

Huff, Joyce L. "'Fattening' Literary History." *Fat Studies: An Interdisciplinary Journal of Body Weight and Society* 2, no. 1 (2013): 30-44.

Hutchins, Loraine. "Letter: And Response." *Off Our Backs* 15, no. 8 (1985): 34.

Hutchins, Loraine. "Review: Shadow on a Tightrope: Writings by Women on Fat Oppression by Lisa Schoenfielder and Barb Wieser." *Off Our Backs* 15, no. 3 (1985): 24-25.

ISAA. "International Size Acceptance Association." http://www.size-acceptance.org/.

Isin, Engin F. "Citizenship in Flux: The Figure of the Activist Citizen." *Subjectivity*. no. 29 (2009): 367-88.

Jackson, Cath. "Fast Food Feminism." *Trouble and Strife* 7 (1985): 39-44.

Jackson, Cath and Rachael Field. "Broadening Out." *Trouble & Strife*. no. 23 (1992): 18-23.

Jagose, Annamarie. *Queer Theory*. Melbourne: Melbourne University Press, 1996.

Janesdaughter, Elly. "Letter: Fatophobic Feminists." *Off Our Backs* 9, no. 7 (1979): 28.

Jeffreys, Sheila. *Beauty and Misogyny: Harmful Cultural Practices in the West*. London: Routledge, 2005.

Jenkins, Tina and Margot Farnham. "As I Am." *Trouble & Strife* 13 (1988).

Jenkins, Tina and Heather Smith. "Fat Liberation." *Spare Rib* 182 (1987): 14-18.

Johnson, Carol A. *Self-Esteem Comes in All Sizes: How to Be Happy and Healthy at Your Natural Weight*. Carlsbad, CA: Gürze Books, 2001.

Johnson, Susan, Devra, Selena, and April. "The Sa/Me Debate." *FaT GiRL* 4 (1995): 8-9.

Johnston, Josée and Judith Taylor. "Feminist Consumerism and Fat Activists: A Comparative Study of Grassroots Activism and the Dove Real Beauty Campaign." *Signs: Journal of Women in Culture and Society* 33, no. 4 (2008): 941-66.

Jonas, Steve. *Just the Weigh You Are: How to Be Fit and Healthy, Whatever*

Your Size. New York: Houghton Mifflin, 1997.

Jones, Karen W. "Naafa Newsletter: Fat and Female–One Woman's View." www.eskimo.com/~largesse/Archives/Fatfemale.html.

Jones, Substantia. "The Adipositivity Project." http://www.adipositivity.com/.

——— "Fatpeopleflippingyouoff." http://fatpeopleflippingyouoff.tumblr. com/.

——— "Smilesizeist." http://smilesizeist.tumblr.com/.

Kacenjar, Rachel. *Free for Chubbies: A Fatshionista's Mini Guide to Repurposing and Reshaping Clothing [Zine].* Cleveland, OH2008. zine.

Kahn, Jeffrey P., Anna C. Mastroiannim and Jeremy Sugarman, eds. *Beyond Consent: Seeking Justice in Research.* Oxford: Oxford University Press, 1998.

Kai-Cheong Chan, Nathan and Allison C. Gillick. "Fatness as a Disability: Questions of Personal and Group Identity." *Disability & Society* 24, no. 2 (2009): 231-43.

Kaplan, Caren. *Questions of Travel: Postmodern Discourses of Displacement.* Durham, NC: Duke University Press, 1996.

Kargbo, Majida. "Toward a New Relationality: Digital Photography, Shame, and the Fat Subject." *Fat Studies: An Interdisciplinary Journal of Body Weight and Society* 2, no. 2 (2013): 160-72.

Katsiaficas, George. "Reading Signs of Change: Social Movement Cultures 1960s to Now." In *Signs of Change.* Edited by Dara Greenwald and Josh MacPhee. 16-21. Oakland and New York: AK Press/Exit Art, 2010.

Kent, Le'a. "Fighting Abjection: Representing Fat Women." In *Bodies out of Bounds: Fatness and Transgression*. Edited by Braziel, Jana Evans and Kathleen LeBesco. 130-50. Los Angeles: University of California Press, 2001.

Kinzel, Lesley. *Two Whole Cakes: How to Stop Dieting and Learn to Love Your Body*. New York: The Feminist Press, 2012.

Kirkland, Anna. *Fat Rights: Dilemmas of Difference and Personhood*. New York: New York University Press, 2008.

Klein, Richard. *Eat Fat*. New York: Pantheon Books, 1996.

Koppelman, Susan, ed. *The Strange History of Suzanne Lafleshe (and Other Stories of Women and Fatness)*. New York: The Feminist Press at the City University of New York, 2003.

Kosofsky Sedgwick, Eve. "Axiomatic." In *Queer Theory*. Edited by Iain Morland and Annabelle Willox. 81-95. Basingstoke: Palgrave Macmillan, 2005.

——— *Epistemology of the Closet*. Berkeley and Los Angeles: University of California Press, 1990.

Krudas Cubensi. "Krudas Cubensi." http://www.krudascubensi.com/.

Kulick, Don and Anne Meneley. *Fat: The Anthopology of an Obsession*. London: Penguin, 2005.

Kunze, Peter C. "Send in the Clowns: Extraordinary Male Protagonists in Contemporary American Fiction." *Fat Studies: An Interdisciplinary Journal of Body Weight and Society* 2, no. 1 (2013): 17-29.

Kwan, Samantha. "Framing the Fat Body: Contested Meanings between

Government, Activists, and Industry." *Sociological Inquiry* 79, no. 1 (2009): 25-50.

Lamm, Nomy. *I'm So Fucking Beautiful [Zine]*. Olympia, WA. 1994.

Land, J. "Pacifica's Wbai: Free Radio and the Claims of Community." *Jump Cut* 41 (1997): 93-101.

Laura. "Gorda!" http://gordazine.tumblr.com/.

Laurel, Alicia Bay. *Living on the Earth*. New York: Vintage Books, Random House, 1971.

LeBesco, Kathleen. *Revolting Bodies: The Struggle to Redefine Fat Identity*. Amherst, MA: University of Massachusetts Press, 2004.

——— "Queering Fat Bodies/Politics." In *Bodies out of Bounds: Fatness and Transgression*. Edited by Braziel, Jana Evans and Kathleen LeBesco. 74-87. Los Angeles: University of California Press, 2001.

Lee, Diana. "Dot Nelson-Turnier: Nolose Woman for the New Millennium." http://www.nolose.org/old/Newsletter/nolose10.html.

——— "In the Beginning... ." http://www.nolose.org/old/Events/2000_Conference/conference_2000.html.

Lee, Shannon. *Fatty Fashions [Zine]*. 2006.

Leland, Andrew. "Elana Dykewomon: An Oral History." Oakland Museum of Calfornia. http://museumca.org/theoaklandstandard/elana-dykewomon-oral-history.

Lepoff, Laurie Ann, Terre Poppe and Fat Sister's. "The Fats of Life: Reflections on the Tyranny of Fatophobia." *Off Our Backs* 13, no. 3 (1983): 30-32.

Lizard, Helen and Shan. "Letter: Thin Thinking." *Off Our Backs* 9, no. 5 (1979): 28.

London Fat Women's Group. "Fat Women's Conference." *Spare Rib*, no. 193 (1988): 54.

Louderback, Llewellyn. *Fat Power*. New York: Hawthorn Books, 1970.

Louderback, Lew. Personal Correspondence with Author, 20 August 2008.

——— "More People Should Be Fat." *Saturday Evening Post*, 4 November 1967, 10-12.

——— *Pretty Boy, Baby Face - I Love You*. Philadelphia: Coronet, 1969.

——— 20 August 2008.

——— *Operation Moon Rocket [Pseudonym Nick Carter]*. London: Tandem, 1968.

Ludenz, Homo. *At the Jungle Gym*. Berlin: Homo Ludenz, n.d. Zine.

Lupton, Deborah. *Fat*. Abingdon: Routledge, 2012.

Lyons, Pat and Debby Burgard. *Great Shape: The First Fitness Guide for Large Women*. Authors Guild Backinprint.com ed. Palo Alto, CA: Bull Publishing Company, 1990.

M@CE. *Venus Envy [Zine]*. Venus Envy. Terre Haute, IN. 1993.

Mabel-Lois, Lynn. "Fat Dykes Don't Make It." *Lesbian Tide* 4, no. 3 (1974): 11.

Manchester Fat Women's Group. "Manchester Fat Women's Group." *Spare Rib*, no. 203 (1989): 57.

Manigault-Bryant, LeRhonda S. "Fat Spirit: Obesity, Religion, and Sapphmammibel in Contemporary Black Film." *Fat Studies: An Interdisciplinary Journal of Body Weight and Society* 2, no. 1 (2013): 56-69.

Maor, Maya. "The Body That Does Not Diminish Itself: Fat Acceptance in Israel's Lesbian Queer Communities." *Journal of Lesbian Studies* 16, no. 2 (2012): 177-98.

Marchessault, Gail, Kevin Thiele, Eleeta Armit, Gwen E. Chapman, Ryna Levy-Milne and Susan I. Barr. "Canadian Dietitians' Understanding of Non-Dieting Approaches in Weight Management." *Canadian Journal of Dietetic Practice and Research* 68, no. 2 (2007): 67-72.

Marla, Glenn. "Mister Marla." http://mistermarla.com/.

Martin, Daniel D. "From Appearance Tales to Oppression Tales: Frame Alignment and Organizational Identity." *Journal of Contemporary Ethnography* 31, no. 2 (2002): 158-206.

Martin, Deborah G., Susan Hanson and Danielle Fontaine. "What Counts as Activism? The Role of Individuals in Creating Change." *Women's Studies Quarterly* 35, no. 3&4 (2007): 78-94.

Mason-John, Valerie. "Keeping up Appearances: The Body and Eating Habits." In *Assaults on Convention: Essays on Lesbian Transgressors.* Edited by Nicola Godwin, Belinda Hollows and Sheridan Nye. 64-79. London: Cassell, 1996.

Mass, Lawrence D. "Bears and Health." In *The Bear Book II: Further Readings in the History and Evolution of a Gay Male Subculture.* Edited by Les K. Wright. 15-37. New York: Haworth Press, 2001.

Matrix. *Embracing Our Beauty, Claiming Our Space: Voices of Fat Liberation.* Santa Cruz, CA: Matrix, 1987.

Maxey, Ian. "Beyond Boundaries? Activism, Academia, Reflexivity and Research." *Area* 31, no. 3 (1999): 199-208.

Mayer, Vivian F. "Foreword." In *Shadow on a Tightrope: Writings by Women on Fat Oppression*. Edited by Schoenfielder, Lisa and Barb Wieser. ix-xvii. Iowa City: Aunt Lute, 1983.

McAfee, Lynn and Miriam Berg. "Advocacy." In *Weight Bias: Nature, Consequences and Remedies*. Edited by Brownell, Kelly D., Leslie Rudd, Marlene B. Schwartz and Rebecca M. Puhl. 285-93. New York: The Guilford Press, 2005.

McAleer, Paul. "Weight Watchers Co-Opts Our Language." http://www.bigfatblog.com/weight-watchers-co-opts-our-language.

McAllister, Heather. "Embodying Fat Liberation." In *The Fat Studies Reader*. Edited by Rothblum, Esther and Sondra Solovay. 305-10. New York: New York University Press, 2009.

McCormack, Heather. "Fat Activism and Body Positivity: Zines for Transforming the Status Quo." *Library Journal*. http://reviews.libraryjournal.com/2012/03/collection-development/zines/fat-activism-and-body-positivity-zines-for-transforming-the-status-quo/.

McKechnie, Rosemary and Barbara Körner. "Unruly Narratives: Discovering the Active Self." In *Narrative, Memory and Identities*. Edited by Robinson, David, Pamela Fisher, Tracey Yeadon-Lee, Sara Jane Robinson and Pete Woodcock. 67-75. Huddersfield: University of Huddersfield, 2009.

McRuer, Robert. *Crip Theory: Cultural Signs of Queerness and Disability*. New York: New York University Press, 2006.

Meleo-Erwin, Zoë. "Disrupting Normal: Toward the 'Ordinary and

Familiar' in Fat Politics." *Feminism & Psychology* 22, no. 3 (2012): 1-15.

———— "Queering the Linkages and Divergences: The Relationship between Fatness and Disability and the Hope for a Livable World." In *Queering Fat Embodiment*. Edited by Cat Pausé, Jackie Wykes and Samantha Murray. 97-114. Farnham: Ashgate, 2014.

———— "Fat Bodies, Qualitative Research and the Spirit of Participatory Action Research." *International Review of Qualitative Research* 3, no. 3 (2010): 335-50.

Millar, Ruth. "A Review of Shadow on a Tightrope: Writings by Woman on Fat Oppression, Edited by Lisa Schoenfielder & Barb Wieser, Aunt Lute Book Company, U.S.A., 1983, Available in the U.K. At £6.95." *Gossip: A Journal of Lesbian Feminist Ethics* 4 (1987): 44-50.

Millman, Marcia. *Such a Pretty Face: Being Fat in America*. Toronto: Norton, 1980.

Misztal, Barbara A. *Theories of Social Remembering*. Maidenhead: Open University Press, 2003.

Mitchell, Allyson. *Ladies Sasquatch*. Hamilton, Ontario: McMaster Museum of Art, 2009.

———— "Pissed Off." In *Fat: The Anthropology of an Obsession*. Edited by Kulick, Don and Anne Meneley. 211-25. London: Penguin, 2005.

Mitchell, Lynnette. "Skinny Lizzie Strikes Back: An Apologia for Thin Women's Liberation." *Gossip: A Journal of Lesbian Feminist Ethics* 3 (1986): 40-44.

Mo'Nique and S.A. McGee. *Skinny Women Are Evil: Notes of a Big Girl in a Small-Minded World*. New York: Atria Books, 2004.

Mobley, Jennifer-Scott. "Tennessee Williams' Ravenous Women: Fat Behavior Onstage." *Fat Studies: An Interdisciplinary Journal of Body Weight and Society* 1, no. 1 (2012): 75-90.

Mollow, Anna. "D isability Studies Gets Fat." *Hypatia* 30, 1 (2015): 199–216.

Monbiot, George. "Obesity Is an Incurable Disease. So Why Is the Government Intent on Punishing Sufferers?" *The Guardian*. http://www.theguardian.com/commentisfree/2015/aug/11/obesity-incurable-disease-cameron-punishing-sufferers.

Moon, Michael and Eve Kosofsky Sedgwick. "Divinity: A Dossier, a Performance Piece, a Little-Understood Emotion." In *Tendencies*. Edited by Eve Kosofsky Sedgwick. 211-46. Durham, NC: Duke University Press, 1994.

Moral. "Letter: Fat Save Species." *Off Our Backs* 10, no. 3 (1980): 31.

Moran, Kate. "One Step Forward, Two Steps Back: Fat Liberation and Overeaters Anonymous." In *Dossier: Oppression De La Grosseur*. Edited by Danielle Charest, Johane Coulombe and Louise Turcotte. 103-12. Montréal: Amazones d'Hier, Lesbiennes d'Aujourdhui, 1992.

Morland, Iain and Annabelle Willox. *Queer Theory*. Basingstoke: Palgrave Macmillan, 2005.

Mulhall, Anne. "Camping up the Emerald Aisle: Queerness in Irish Popular Culture." In *Irish Postmodernisms and Popular Culture*. Edited by Wanda Balzano, Anne Mulhall and Moynagh Sullivan. 210-19. Basingstoke: Palgrave Macmillan, 2007.

Munter, Carol. "Fat and the Fantasy of Perfection." In *Pleasure and Danger: Exploring Female Sexuality*. Edited by Carole S. Vance. 225-31.

London: Pandora Press, 1992.

Murray, Samantha. *The 'Fat' Female Body*. Basingstoke: Palgrave Macmillan, 2008.

———— "'Banded Bodies': The Somatechnics of Gastric Banding." In *Somatechnics: Queering the Technologisation of Bodies*. Edited by Nikki Sullivan and Samantha Murray. 153-70. Farnham: Ashgate, 2009.

———— "(Un/Be)Coming Out? Rethinking Fat Politics." *Social Semiotics* 15, no. 2 (2005): 153-63.

———— "Women under/in Control? Embodying Eating after Gastric Banding." *Radical Psychology* 8, no. 1 (2009).

NAAFA. "Naafa Online." http://www.naafaonline.com/.

———— "Naafa's Official Position: Weight-Loss Surgery." http://www.naafaonline.com/dev2/about/doc-weightLossSurgery.html.

Nanfeldt, Suzan. *The Plus-Size Guide to Looking Great*. New York: Plume, 1996.

Naples, Nancy A. and Karen Bojar. *Teaching Feminist Activism: Strategies from the Field*. New York: Routledge, 2002.

Narby, Caroline and Katherine Phelps. "As Big as a House: Representations of the Extremely Fat Woman and the Home." *Fat Studies: An Interdisciplinary Journal of Body Weight and Society* 2, no. 2 (2013): 147-59.

Nash, Hugh, ed. *Progress as If Survival Mattered. A Handbook for a Conserver Society*. San Francisco: Friends of the Earth, 1977.

Nelson, Marjory. "Letter: Thinly Veiled Insult." *Off Our Backs* 13, no. 5 (1983): 30.

Nelson-Turnier, Dot. "Notes from the Founder." http://www.nolose.org/old/Newsletter/nolose02.html.

——— "Why a National Organization for Lesbians of Size?" http://www.nolose.org/old/Newsletter/nolose01.html.

Nichols, Grace. *The Fat Black Woman's Poems*. London: Virago, 1984.

Nimoy, Leonard. *The Full Body Project: Photographs by Leonard Nimoy*. Minneapolis: Consortium, 2007.

NOLOSE. "Nolose.Org." http://www.nolose.org.

Norimitsu, Onishi. "Japan, Seeking Trim Waists, Measures Millions." *New York Times*. http://www.nytimes.com/2008/06/13/world/asia/13fat.html?_r=1&scp=1&sq=japanese%20government%20measure%20waist&st=cse&oref=slogin.

O'Shaughnessy, Sara and Emily Huddart Kennedy. "Relational Activism: Reimagining Women's Environmental Work as Cultural Change." *Canadian Journal of Sociology/Cahiers Canadiens de Sociologie* 35, no. 4 (2010): 551-72.

Obesity Action Coalition. "Obesity Action Coalition." www.obesityaction.org/.

Ochterski, Jean. "There Are No Fat People in the Netherlands: Embodied Identities, Hypervisibility, and the Contextual Relevancy of Fatness." In *Independent Study Project (ISP) Collection*. South Hadley, MA: Mount Holyoke College, 2013.

Off Our Backs. *Off Our Backs: Body Image.* Vol. 34. Arlington, VA: Off Our Backs, 2004.

Oliver, J. Eric. *Fat Politics: The Real Story Behind America's Obesity Epidemic.* New York: Oxford University Press US, 2006.

Orbach, Susie. *Fat Is a Feminist Issue: How to Lose Weight Permanently –without Dieting.* London: Arrow Books, 1978.

——— *Bodies.* London: Profile Books, 2009.

——— *Fat Is a Feminist Issue 2: How to Free Yourself from Feeling Obsessive About Food.* London: Hamlyn, 1982.

Orbach, Susie and Compulsive Eating Supervision Study Group at The Women's Therapy Centre. "Responses to Nicky Diamond." *Feminist Review* 21 (1985): 119-22.

Otobong, Karis. "Fattened by Force." *Trouble & Strife*, no. 23 (1992): 8-9.

Pathé. *Plump and Lovely (Miss Fat and Beautiful Contest) [Video].* London: Pathé, 1962.

Pauly Morgan, Kathryn. "Foucault, Ugly Ducklings, and Technoswans: Analysing Fat Hatred, Weight-Loss Surgery, and Compulsory Biomedicalised Aesthetics in America." *The International Journal of Feminist Approaches to Bioethics* 4, no. 1 (2011): 188-220.

Pausé, Cat. "The Epistemology of Fatness." http://friendofmarilyn. com/2012/04/05/the-epistemology-of-fatness/.

Pausé, Cat. "Causing a Commotion: Queering Fat in Cyberspace." In *Queering Fat Embodiment.* Edited by Cat Pausé, Jackie Wykes and Samatha Murray. 75-88. Farnham: Ashgate, 2014.

———— "X-Static Process: Intersectionality within the Field of Fat Studies." *Fat Studies: An Interdisciplinary Journal of Body Weight and Society* 3, no. 2 (2014): 80-85.

Pausé, Cat, Jackie Wykes and Samantha Murray, eds. *Queering Fat Embodiment*. Farnham: Ashgate, 2014.

Perkins, Natalie. "No Diet Talk; a Badge for Your Blog." http://www. definatalie.com/2011/11/18/no-diet-talk-a-badge-for-your-blog/.

Peterson, Latoya. "Intersectionality Extends to Fat Acceptance Too!" *Racialicious*. http://www.racialicious.com/2008/03/24/intersectionality-extends-to-fat-acceptance-too/.

Phillipson, Andrea. "Re-Reading 'Lipoliteracy': Putting Emotions to Work in Fat Studies Scholarship." *Fat Studies: An Interdisciplinary Journal of Body Weight and Society* 2, no. 1 (2013): 70-86.

Piasecki, Amanda. "Fatshionista." http://community.livejournal.com/fatshionista/.

Pietaro, John. "The Cultural Worker." http://theculturalworker.blogspot.co.uk/2010/12/communist-cultural-workers-brief.html.

Polack, Devra. "Queer Punks Chew the Fat." *FaT GiRL* 6 (1996): 6-7.

Pollard, Diana. "Beyond Fat Liberation: Towards a Celebration of Size Diversity." In *Sizeable Reflections: Big Women Living Full Lives*. Edited by Shelley Bovey. 22-37. London: The Women's Press, 2000.

———— *Freesize*. Vol. 3, London. 1999.

Polletta, Francesca. "Contending Stories: Narrative in Social Movements." *Qualitative Sociology* 21, no. 4 (1998): 419-46.

Poretsky, Golda. *Stop Dieting Now: 25 Reasons to Stop, 25 Ways to Heal.* Astoria, NY: Body Love Wellness, 2010.

Post, Steve. *Playing in the Fm Band: A Personal Account of Free Radio.* New York: The Viking Press, 1974.

Probyn, Elspeth. "Silences Behind the Mantra: Critiquing Feminist Fat." *Feminism & Psychology* 18, no. 3 (2008): 401-04.

Prohaska, Ariane. "Help Me Get Fat! Feederism as Communal Deviance on the Internet." *Deviant Behavior* 35 (2014): 263–74.

Puar, Jasbir K. *Terrorist Assemblages: Homonationlism in Queer Times.* Durham, NC: Duke University Press, 2007.

Pyle, Nathaniel C. and Michael I. Loewy. "Double Stigma: Fat Men and Their Male Admirers." In *The Fat Studies Reader.* Edited by Esther Rothblum and Sondra Solovay. 143-50. New York: New York University Press, 2009.

Rage, Raju and Mîran N. "Time Travelling Brown Bears: Intergenerational Interviews with Two Transmasculine Femmes of Color on Healing Justice." https://heimatkunde.boell.de/2013/05/01/time-travelling-brown-bears-intergenerational-interviews-two-transmasculine-femmes-color.

RationalWiki. "Fat Acceptance Movement." http://rationalwiki.org/wiki/Fat_acceptance_movement.

Ratliffe, Jamie. "Drawing on Burlesque: Excessive Display and Fat Desire in the Work of Cristina Vela." *Fat Studies: An Interdisciplinary Journal of Body Weight and Society* 2, no. 2 (2013): 118-31.

Reay-Smith, Philip. "The World's First Lesbian Beauties." *The Pink Paper,* 4 July 1997.

Reddit. "Removing Harassing Subreddits." http://np.reddit.com/r/announcements/comments/39bpam/removing_harassing_subreddits/.

Reed-Danahay, Deborah E. *Auto/Ethnography: Rewriting the Self and the Social*. Oxford: Berg, 1997.

Relly, J.E. "The Big Issue." http://www.tucsonweekly.com/tw/10-01-98/feat.htm.

Rensenbrink, Greta. "Fat's No Four-Letter Word: Fat Feminism and Identity Politics in the 1970s and 1980s." In *Historicizing Fat in Anglo-American Culture*. Edited by Elena Levy-Navarro. 213-43. Columbus, OH: The Ohio State University Press, 2010.

Retter, Yolanda. "Lesbian Activism in Los Angeles, 1970-1979." In *Queer Frontiers: Millennial Geographies, Genders, and Generations*. Edited by Joseph Allen Boone. 196-221. Madison, WI The University of Wisconsin Press, 2000.

Riggs, Cynthia. "Fat Women and Clothing: An Interview with Judy Freespirit." In *Shadow on a Tightrope: Writings by Women on Fat Oppression*. Edited by Lisa Schoenfielder and Barb Wieser. 139-43. Iowa City: Aunt Lute, 1983.

Riot, Wyatt. "Wyatt Riot." http://www.originalplumbing.com/index.php/team/itemlist/user/507-wyattriot.

Roark, Deb. "Letter: Sized up &Boxed In." *Off Our Backs* 6, no. 5 (1976): 30.

Roberts, Nancy. *Breaking All the Rules: Looking Good and Feeling Great No Matter What Your Size*. London: Penguin, 1987.

Robertson Textor, Alex. "Organisation, Specialisation, and Desires in the Big

Men's Movement: Preliminary Research in the Study of Subculture-Formation." *Journal of Gay, Lesbian, and Bisexual Identity* 4, no. 3 (1999): 217-39.

Robison, Jon. "Health at Every Size: Toward a New Paradigm of Weight and Health." *Medscape General Medicine* 7, no. 3 (2005): 13.

Robison, Jon, Kelly Putnam, and Laura McKibbin. "Health at Every Size: A Compassionate, Effective Approach for Helping Individuals with Weight-Related Concerns—Part I." *American Association of Occupational Health Nurses Journal* 55, no. 4 (2007): 143-50.

Rochman, Bonnie. "Do I Look Fat? Don't Ask. A Campaign to Ban 'Fat Talk.'" *Time Inc.* http://www.time.com/time/nation/article/0,8599,2025345,00.html.

Rogge, Mary Madeline and Marti Greenwald. "Obesity, Stigma, and Civilized Oppression." *Advances in Nursing Science* 27, no. 4 (2004): 301-15.

Rose, Nikolas. *Powers of Freedom: Reframing Political Thought.* Cambridge: Cambridge University Press, 1999.

Rothblum, Esther and Sondra Solovay. *The Fat Studies Reader.* New York: New York University Press, 2009.

Rothblum, Esther D. "Commentary: Lesbians Should Take the Lead in Removing the Stigma That Has Long Been Associated with Body Weight." *Psychology of Sexual Orientation and Gender Diversity* (2014): 1-6.

——— "Why a Journal on Fat Studies?" *Fat Studies: An Interdisciplinary Journal of Body Weight and Society* 1, no. 1 (2012): 3-5.

Rotunda Press. "Watchout Rotunda Is Coming!" *Spare Rib*, no. 211 (1990): 54.

Rubin, Gayle. "Thinking Sex: Notes for a Radical Theory of the Politics of Sexuality." In *Pleasure and Danger*. Edited by Carole Vance. 267-319. Boston: Routledge & Keegan Paul, 1984.

Rubin, Jerry. *Do It! Scenarios of the Revolution*. New York: Simon and Schuster, 1970.

Russel Hochschild, Arlie. *The Managed Heart: Commercialisation of Human Feeling*. Berkeley and Los Angeles: University of California Press, 2003.

Russell, Shannon. "Shut Down." http://fiercefatties.com/2012/03/22/shut-down/.

Rygh Glen, Lily. "Big Trouble: Are Eating Disorders the Lavender Menace of the Fat Acceptance Movement?" *Bitch Magazine: Feminist Response to Pop Culture* 38 (2008): 40-45.

Saguy, Abigail. "Sex, Inequality, and Ethnography: Response to Erich Goode." *Qualitative Sociology* 25, no. 4 (2002): 549-556.

———*What's Wrong with Fat?* New York: Oxford University Press, 2014.

Saguy, Abigail C. and Kevin W. Riley. "Weighing Both Sides: Morality, Mortality, and Framing Contests over Obesity." *Journal of Health Politics, Policy & Law* 30, no. 5 (2005): 869-921.

Saguy, Abigail C. and Anna Ward. "Coming out as Fat: Rethinking Stigma." *Social Psychology Quarterly* 74 (2011): 53-75.

Said, Edward W. *Orientalism*. New York: Pantheon Books, 1978.

——— *The World, the Text, and the Critic*. Cambridge, MA: Harvard University Press, 1983.

Sayer, Andrew. "Misecognition: The Unequal Division of Labour and Contributive Justice." In *The Politics of Misrecognition*. Edited by Simon Thompson and Majid Yar. 87-104. Farnham: Ashgate, 2011.

Scaraboto, Daiane and Eileen Fischer. "Frustrated Fatshionistas: An Institutional Theory Perspective on Consumer Quests for Greater Choice in Mainstream Markets." *Journal of Consumer Research* 39, no.6 (2013): 1234-1257.

Scaraboto, Daiane and Severino Joaquim Nunes Pereira. "Rhetorical Strategies of Consumer Activists: Reframing Market Offers to Promote Change." *Brazilian Administration review* 10, no. 4 (2013): 389-414.

Schoenfielder, Lisa and Barb Wieser. *Shadow on a Tightrope: Writings by Women on Fat Oppression*. San Francisco: Aunt Lute, 1983.

Schorb, Friedrich. "Fat Politics in Europe: Theorizing on the Premises and Outcomes of European Anti-'Obesity-Epidemic' Policies." *Fat Studies: An Interdisciplinary Journal of Body Weight and Society* 2, no. 1 (2013): 3-16.

Schulman, Sarah. *The Gentrification of the Mind: Witness to a Lost Imagination*. Oakland, CA: University of California Press, 2012.

Schwartz, Hillel. *Never Satisfied: A Cultural History of Diets, Fantasies and Fat*. New York: The Free Press, 1986.

Secomb, Linnell. "Fractured Community." *Hypatia* 15, no. 2 (2000): 133-50.

Seligman, Martin. *Learned Optimism: How to Change Your Mind and Your Life*. New York: Knopf, 1991.

Shanker, Wendy. *The Fat Girl's Guide to Life*. New York: Bloomsbury, 2005.

Shaw, Andrea Elizabeth. *The Embodiment of Disobedience: Fat Black Women's Unruly Political Bodies*. Lanham, MD: Lexington Books, 2006.

Sheffield, Shirley. "Padded Lillies." http://paddedlilies.com/.

Sherman Heyl, Barbara. "Ethnographic Interviewing." In *Handbook of Ethnography*. Edited by Paul Atkinson, Amanda Coffey, Sara Delamont, John Lofland and Lyn Lofland. 369-83. London: SAGE, 2001.

Shilling, Chris. *The Body and Social Theory*. 2nd ed. London: SAGE, 1993.

Shuai, Tara. "A Different Kind of Fat Rant: People of Color and the Fat Acceptance Movement." http://web.archive.org/web/20080919002110/http://www.fatshionista.com/cms/index.php?option=com_content&task=view&id=180&Itemid=9

Shuai, Tara, Galadriel Mozee, Virgie Tovar, Geleni Fontaine, Margarita Feminista, Julia Starkey, Amy Ongiri, M. Taueret Davis and Naima Lowe. "A Response to White Fat Activism from People of Color in the Fat Justice Movement." NOLOSE. http://www.nolose.org/activism/POC.php.

Shuai, Tara, Galadriel Mozee, Kim Paulus, Rachel, Geleni Fontaine, Abby Weintraub, Jen Herrington, Joe, Sondra, Zoe. "Nolose Policy Change: Inclusion and Moving from Identity to Intention." http://www.nolose.org/11/genderpolicy.php.

Shugart, Helene A. "Consuming Citizen: Neoliberating the Obese Body." *Communication, Culture & Critique* 3 (2010): 105-26.

Silverstone, Catherine. "Duckie's Gay Shame: Critiquing Pride and Selling Shame in Club Performance." *Contemporary Theatre Review* 22, no. 1 (2012): 62-78.

Simic, Zora. "Fat as a Feminist Issue: A History." In *Fat Sex: New Directions in Theory and Activism*. Edited by Helen Hester and Caroline Walters. 15-35. Farnham: Ashgate, 2015.

Skeggs, Bev. *Class, Self, Culture*. London: Routledge, 2004.

———— *Formations of Class & Gender*. London: SAGE, 1997.

Skrabanek, Petr. *The Death of Humane Medicine and the Rise of Coercive Healthism*. Bury St Edmonds: The Social Affairs Unit, 1994.

Smailes, Sophie. "Negotiating and Navigating My Fat Body–Feminist Autoethnographic Encounters." *Athenea Digital* 14, no. 1 (2014): 49-61.

Smith, Carolyn. "Under the Radar: Fat Activism and the London 2012 Olympics, an Interview with Charlotte Cooper." http://www.gamesmonitor.org.uk/node/1647.

Smith, Heather. "Creating a Politics of Appearance." *Trouble & Strife* 16, no. Summer (1989): 36-41.

Smith, Linda Tuhiwai. *Decolonizing Methodologies: Research and Indigenous Peoples*. London: Zed Books, 1999.

Snider, Stefanie. "Fatness and Visual Culture: A Brief Look at Some Contemporary Projects." *Fat Studies: An Interdisciplinary Journal of Body Weight and Society* 1, no. 1 (2012): 13-31.

———— "Revisioning Fat Lesbian Subjects in Contemporary Lesbian Periodicals." *Journal of Lesbian Studies* 14, no. 2 (2010): 174-84.

Sobal, Jeffrey and Donna Maurer. *Interpreting Weight: The Social Management of Fatness and Thinness*. Edison, NJ: Aldine Transaction, 1999.

———— *Weighty Issues: Fatness and Thinness as Social Problems*. Edison, NJ: Aldine Transaction, 1999.

Solovay, Sondra. "Remedies for Weight-Based Discrimination." In *Weight Bias: Nature, Consequences and Remedies*, edited by K. D.; Brownell, Rebecca M.; Puhl, Marlene B.; Schwartz and Leslie Rudd, 212-22. New York: The Guilford Press, 2005.

———— *Tipping the Scales of Justice: Fighting Weight-Based Discrimination*. Amherst, NY: Prometheus Books, 2000.

Soncrant, Jean and Lynn McAfee. "Airline Tips for Large Passengers." *Healthy Weight Journal* 15, no. 4 (2001): 63.

Spivak, Gayatri Chakravorty. *In Other Worlds: Essays in Cultural Politics*. New York: Routledge, 1987.

Spry, Tami. "Performing Autoethnography: An Embodied Methodological Praxis." In *Emergent Methods in Social Research*. Edited by Sharlene Nagy Hesse-Biber and Patricia Leavy. 183-211. Thousand Oaks, CA: SAGE, 2006.

Stanley, Eric A. and Nat Smith. *Captive Genders: Trans Embodiment and the Prison Industrial Complex*. Edinburgh: AK Press, 2011.

Stein, Judith. "Fat Liberation: No Losers Here." *Sojourner* 6, no. 9 (1981): 8.

———— *Fat Oppression and Fat Liberation: Some Basic Ideas*. Boston1980.

———— "Get Your Foot Off My Neck: Fat Liberation." *Gay Community News*, 28 June 1986, 6.

———— *The New Haven Fat Women's Health Conference: Proceedings of the First Feminist Fat Activists' Working Meeting*. New Haven, CT: Fat

Liberator Publications, 1980. Largesse Fat Liberation Archives.

——— "On Getting Strong: Notes from a Fat Woman, in Two Parts." In *Shadow on a Tightrope: Writings by Women on Fat Oppression*. Edited by Lisa Schoenfielder and Barb Wieser. 106-10. Iowa City: Aunt Lute, 1983.

Stein, Judith A. and Beryl-Elise Hoffstein. *Proceedings of the First Feminist Fat Activists' Working Meeting: April 18-20, 1980, New Haven, Ct*. Minneapolis, MN: Fat Liberator Publications, 1980.

Stein, Judith and Meridith Lawrence. *30 Big Minutes with Fat Liberation [Radio]*. Boston: Massachusetts Institute of Technology, 1985.

——— *Plain Talk About Fat [Radio]*. Boston: Massachusetts Institute of Technology, 1984.

Stein, Judith, ReaRea Sears, Pam Mitchell, Robin Newmark and Jennifer Purnell. "The Political History of Fat Liberation: An Interview." *The Second Wave* 3 (1981): 32-37.

Stimson, Karen. "Fat Feminist Herstory, 1969-1993: A Personal Memoir." http://www.eskimo.com/~largesse/Archives/herstory.html.

——— *The Fat Underground: The Original Radical Fat Feminists-a Commemorative Sourcebook from the Archives of Largesse, the Network for Size Esteem*. New Haven, CT: Largesse, 1995.

Stinson, Susan. *Fat Girl Dances with Rocks*. New York: Spinsters Ink, 1994.

——— "Fat Girls Need Fiction." In *The Fat Studies Reader*. Edited by Esther Rothblum and Sondra Solovay. 231-34. New York: New York University Press, 2009.

——— *Martha Moody*. London: The Women's Press, 1996.

——— "Speakout against Fat Hatred." *Healthy Weight Journal* 14, no. 4 (2000): 62.

——— "Belly Song." *Sinister Wisdom* 32 (1987): 111-13.

——— *Belly Songs: In Celebration of Fat Women.* Northampton, MA: Susan Stinson, 1993. Chap Book.

———"Nothing Succeeds Like Excess: Corporate Greed Goes Unchecked in a Fat-Phobic Society." *The Women's Review of Books* XVIII, no. 10-11 (2001): 16.

———*Venus of Chalk.* Ann Arbor, MI: Firebrand Books, 2004.

——— "Whole Cloth." *Common Lives/Lesbian Lives* 19 (1986): 58-61.

Stockwell, Rita. "Letter: Shadow-Boxing." *Off Our Backs* 15, no. 8 (1985): 34.

Stone, Shira. "Speaking out, Reaching Out." http://www.nolose.org/old/Newsletter/nolose04.html.

Stone-Mediatore, Shari. *Reading Across Borders: Storytelling and Knowledges of Resistance.* New York: Palgrave Macmillan, 2003.

Stryker, Kitty. "Fat Sex Works!" In *Hot & Heavy: Fierce Fat Girls on Life, Love & Fashion.* Edited by Virgie Tovar Berkeley. CA: Seal Press, 2012.

Sturgis, Susanna J. "Is This the New Thing We're Going to Have to Be P.C. About?" *Sinister Wisdom* 28 (1985): 16-47.

Sturmer, Stefan, Bernd Simon, Michael Loewy and Heike Jorger. "The Dual-Pathway Model of Social Movement Participation: The Case of the Fat Acceptance Movement." *Social Psychology Quarterly* 66, no. 1

(2003): 71-82.

Sullivan, Nikki. *A Critical Introduction to Queer Theory*. Edinburgh: Edinburgh University Press, 2003.

Sullivan, Nikki and Samantha Murray. *Somatechnics: Queering the Technologisation of Bodies*. Farnham: Ashgate, 2009.

Suresha, Ron. "Bear Roots." In *The Bear Book: Readings in the History and Evolution of a Gay Male Subculture*. Edited by Les K. Wright. 41-49. New York: Harrington Park Press, 1997.

Swarc, Sandy. "Junkfood Science." http://junkfoodscience.blogspot.com/.

Sykes, Heather. *Queer Bodies: Sexualities, Genders, & Fatness in Physical Education*. New York: Peter Lang, 2011.

Taueret and Bunny. *Glutton for Fatshion [Zine]*. New York. 2009.

——— *Glutton for Fatshion #2 [Zine]*. Vol. 2. New York. 2010.

Taylor, Sonya Renee. "The Body Is Not an Apology." http:// thebodyisnotanapology.com/.

Teddern, Sue. "Fat Pride and Prejudice." *The Guardian*, 14 February 1989, 21.

Terra. "Ator Será O Líder Da "Fattylympics", Protesto Contra Os Jogos." Terra Networks Brasil S.A. http://esportes.terra.com.br/jogos-olimpicos/ londres-2012/noticias/0,,OI5877012-EI19410,00-Ator+sera+o+lider+d a+Fattylympics+protesto+contra+os+Jogos.html.

The Fat Underground. *The Fat Underground*. n.d. Video.

———— "Introduction to Fat Underground and Radical Feminist Therapy Collective, from Women's Center Brochure." http://web. archive.org/web/20070808155443/http://www.largesse.net/Archives/ FU/women'scenter.html.

———— "More Women Are on Diets Than in Jail." *Sister* November (1974): 4.

———— *Position Paper: Eating.* Largesse Fat Liberation Archive. Edited by The Fat Underground Los Angeles/ New Haven CT: The Fat Underground/Largesse Fat Liberation Archives, 1974.

———— *Position Paper: Health of Fat Women...The Real Problem.* Largesse Fat Liberation Archives. Edited by The Fat Underground Los Angeles/ New Haven, CT: The Fat Underground/Largesse Fat Liberation Archives, 1974.

———— *Position Paper: Job Discrimination.* Largesse Fat Liberation Archive. Edited by The Fat Underground Los Angeles/New Haven, CT: The Fat Underground/Largesse Fat Liberation Archives, 1974.

———— *Position Paper: Psychiatry.* Largesse Fat Liberation Archives. Edited by The Fat Underground Los Angeles/New Haven, CT: The Fat Underground/Largesse Fat Liberation Archives, 1974.

———— *Position Paper: Sexism.* Largesse Fat Liberation Archives. Edited by The Fat Underground Los Angeles/New Haven, CT: The Fat Underground/Largesse Fat Liberation Archives, 1974.

The Galactic Acetic Acid Liberation Front. "Fat Fear." *Off Our Backs* 9, no. 4 (1979): 18.

The New York Times. "Fat Times in New Haven." http://www.eskimo. com/~largesse/Archives/NYT.html.

Thomas, Samantha, Asuntha Karunaratne, Sophie Lewis, David Castle, Natalie Knoesen, Roberta Honigman, Jim Hyde, Rick Kausman and Paul Komesaroff. "'Just Bloody Fat!': A Qualitative Study of Body Image, Self-Esteem and Coping in Obese Adults." *International Journal of Mental Health Promotion* 12, no. 1 (2010): 39-49.

Throsby, Karen. "'I'd Kill Anyone Who Tried to Take My Band Away': Obesity Surgery, Critical Fat Politics and the 'Problem' of Patient Demand." *Somatechnics* 2, no. 1 (2012): 107-26.

Tillmon, Johnnie. "Welfare as a Women's Issue." *Ms* 1, no. 1 (1972): 111.

Tilly, Charles. *Social Movements, 1768-2004*. Boulder, CO: Paradigm Publishers, 2004.

Tirosh, Yofi. "The Right to Be Fat." *Yale Journal of Health Policy, Law and Ethics* XII, no. 2 (2012): 266-335.

Tomlinson, John. *Cultural Imperialism: A Critical Introduction*. London: Continuum, 1991.

Tomrley, Corinna. "Introduction: Finding the Fat, the Fighting and the Fabulous, Or: The Political, Personal and Pertinent Imperatives of Fsuk." In *Fat Studies in the Uk*. Edited by Corinna Tomrley and Ann Kaloski Naylor. 9-16. York: Raw Nerve, 2009.

Tomrley, Corinna and Ann Kaloski Naylor eds. *Fat Studies in the Uk*. York: Raw Nerve Books, 2009.

Touraine, Alain. "On the Frontier of Social Movements." *Current Sociology* 52, no. 4 (2004): 717-725.

Tovar, Virgie, ed. *Hot & Heavy: Fierce Fat Girls on Life, Love and Fashion*. Berkeley, CA: Seal Press, 2012.

————"Pecan Pie, Sex, and Other Revolutionary Things." In *Hot & Heavy: Fierce Fat Girls on Life, Love & Fashion*. Edited by Virgie Tovar. 167-76. Berkeley, CA: Seal Press, 2012.

Turner, Bryan. *Regulating Bodies: Essays in Medical Sociology*. London: Routledge, 1992.

Turner, Bryan S. *The Body and Society: Explorations in Social Theory*. 2nd ed. London: SAGE, 1996.

Tylka, Tracy L., Rachel A. Annunziato, Deb Burgard, Sigrún Daníelsdóttir, Ellen Shuman, Chad Davis and Rachel M. Calogero. "The Weight-Inclusive Versus Weight-Normative Approach to Health: Evaluating the Evidence for Prioritizing Well-Being over Weight Loss." *Journal of Obesity* 2014 (2014) doi:10.1155/2014/983495.

Unsigned for obvious reasons. "Letter: Fat Kills." *Off Our Backs* 9, no. 7 (1979): 28.

Vale, V. "Fat Girl." In *Zines! Volume One: Incendiary Interviews with Independent Publishers*. Edited by V. Vale. 130-49. San Francisco: Re/Search Publications, 1999.

Valocchi, Steve. "Riding the Crest of a Protest Wave? Collective Action Frames in the Gay Liberation Movement, 1969-1973." *Mobilization: An International Quarterly* 4, no. 1 (1999): 59-73.

van der Ziel, Cornelia and Jacqueline Tourville. *Big, Beautiful, and Pregnant: Expert Advice and Comforting Wisdom for the Expecting Plus-Size Woman*. New York: Marlowe & Co, 2002.

Vannucci, Delfina and Richard Singer. *Come Hell or High Water: A Handbook on Collective Process Gone Awry*. Oakland and Edinburgh: AK Press, 2010.

Vargas, Chris and Greg Youmans. *Falling in Love...with Chris and Greg: Episode 3 - Food!* Oakland, CA, 2010. Digital Video.

Voigts, Ines and Gesine Claus. "Invasion of the Chubsters." *an.schläge* December/January (2010): 20-21.

Voigts, Ines, Gesine Claus and Nina Schulz. "The Chubsters: Interview Mit Charlotte Cooper." *Hugs and Kisses: tender to all gender* 5 (15 October 2009): 52-55.

von Liebenstein, Stephanie. "Confronting Weight Discrimination in Germany–the Foundation of a Fat Acceptance Organization." *Fat Studies: An Interdisciplinary Journal of Body Weight and Society* 1, no. 2 (2012): 166-79.

Vron. "Taking up Space: From Fat Oppression to Fat Liberation." *From the Flames* 4 (1991): 4-13.

Walker, Sarai. *Dietland.* New York: Houghton Mifflin, 2015.

Walters, Suzanna Danuta. "From Here to Queer: Radical Feminism, Postmodernism, and the Lesbian Menace." In *Queer Theory.* Edited by Iain Morland and Annabelle Willox. 6-21. Basingstoke: Palgrave Macmillan, 2005.

Wang, Lucy. "Weight Discrimination: One Size Fits All Remedy?" *Yale Law Journal* 117, no. 8 (2008): 1900-45.

Wann, Marilyn. "1000 Fat Cranes." http://www.myspace.com/1000fatcranes.

———"Fat Crane Video #1." http://www.myspace.com/video/1-000-fat-cranes/fat-crane-video-035-6/40192991#!/video/1000fatcranes/fat-crane-video-035-1/40184296.

——— "I Appreciated Very Much This Post Today from Marianne Kirby on the Rotund and Also Comments There from Julia Starkey, Margarita Femme-Inista, and Others." Facebook. https://www.facebook.com/marilynwann.

Wann, Marilyn. "Apology..." http://istandagainstweightbullying.tumblr.com/.

——— *Fat!So? Because You Don't Have to Apologize for Your Size!* Berkeley CA: Ten Speed Press, 1998.

Wardrop, Alex and Deborah M. Withers, eds. *The Para-Academic Handbook: A Toolkit for Making-Learning-Creating-Acting.* Bristol: HammerOn Press, 2014.

Warin, Megan J. and Jessica S. Gunson. "The Weight of the Word: Knowing Silences in Obesity Research." *Qualitative Health Research* XX, no. X (2013): 1-11.

Warner, Michael. "Queer and Then? The End of Queer Theory?" *The Chronicle of Higher Education.* http://chronicle.com/article/QueerThen-/130161.

Welch, Michael. *Flag Burning: Moral Panic and the Criminalisation of Protest.* New York: Walter de Gruyter, 2000.

Wettergren, Åsa. "Fun and Laughter: Culture Jamming and the Emotional Regime of Late Capitalism." *Social Movement Studies* 8, no. 1 (2009): 1-10.

White, Francis Ray. "Fat, Queer, Dead: 'Obesity' and the Death Drive." *Somatechnics* 2, no. 1 (2012): 1-17.

Whitesel, Jason. *Fat Gay Men: Girth, Mirth, and the Politics of Stigma.* New York: New York University Press, 2014.

Wieviorka, Michel. "After New Social Movements." *Social Movement Studies* 4, no. 1 (2005): 1-19.

WildSister, Katy. "Letter: Not Buying It." *Off Our Backs* 20, no. 8 (1990): 34.

Wiley, Carol. *Journeys to Self-Acceptance: Fat Women Speak*. Freedom, CA: The Crossing Press, 1994.

Wilton, Tamsin. *Good for You: A Handbook of Lesbian Health and Wellbeing*. London: Cassell, 1997.

Withers, Deborah M. "Strategic Affinities: Historiography and Epistemology in Contemporary Feminist Knowledge Politics." *European Journal of Women's Studies* 22, no. 2 (2015): 129-42.

——— "Women's Liberation, Relationships and the 'Vicinity of Trauma'." *Oral History* 40, no. 1 (2012): 79-88.

Wolf, Naomi. *The Beauty Myth*. London: Chatto, 1990.

Wood, Wendy, Sharon Lundgren, Judith A. Ouellette, Shelly Busceme, and Tamela Blackstone. "Minority Influence: A Meta-Analytic Review of Social Influence Processes." *Psychological Bulletin* 115, no. 3 (1994): 323-45.

Woodman, Marion. *The Owl Was a Baker's Daughter: Obesity, Anorexia Nervosa and the Repressed*. Toronto: Inner City Books, 1982.

World Health Organization. *Obesity: Preventing and Managing the Global Epidemic*. Who Technical Report Series 894. Geneva: World Health Organization, 2000.

Wright, Jan and Valerie Harwood. *Biopolitics and the Obesity Epidemic: Governing Bodies*. London: Taylor & Francis, 2008.

www.Ringsurf.com. "Ringsurf: Fat and Proud." http://www.ringsurf.
com/ring/fat_prd/.

Wykes, Jackie. "'I Saw a Knock-Out': Fatness, (in)Visibility, and Desire
in Shallow Hall." *Somatechnics* 2, no. 1 (2012): 60-79.

Yancey, Antronette K., Joanne Leslie and Emily K. Abel. "Obesity at the
Crossroads: Feminist and Public Health Perspectives." *Signs* 31, no. 2
(2006): 425-47.

Zerbe Enns, Carolyn. *Feminist Theories and Feminist Psychotherapies:
Origins, Themes, and Diversity*. Binghampton, NY: Harrington Park
Press, 1997.

INDEX

Lesbisch Schwule Filmtage, 209
Let It All Hang Out, 132
letter writing, 54-55, 182
liveable lives, 2, 82, 94
lived experience, awakening, 15, 80, 97, 103, 217
London, 10, 65, 90, 98, 140-44, 159, 178, 195, 205, 208, 211, 213-14
London Fat Women's Group, 98, 140-44, 61n20
London Women's Centre, 143
looksism, 123
Los Angeles, 69, 116-17, 124-25, 128, 130-31, 159
Louderback, Ann, 111, 115
Louderback, Llewellyn (Lew), 111-13, 115, 120
Love Your Body, 17, 86, 159-60
Lucy, Lady, 206,
Lupton, Deborah, 33, 177n25

Mabel-Lois, Lynn. *See* Lynn McAfee
MacAllister, Heather, 89, 204
maintaining power and status, 25
Making It Big, 132
marginalisation, 5, 7, 14, 23, 31, 34, 37-38, 40, 48, 57, 59, 93, 104, 111, 116, 139, 143, 162, 169, 171, 180, 216
margins, 35, 37, 162, 193, 203, 213
materiality, 86-87
Mayer, Vivian F., 120, 123, 127, 136, 149, 160
McAfee, Lynn, 61n21, 117, 123-25, 134, 200
medicalisation, 1n1, 28, 50, 94, 117, 123-24, 187
Meleo-Erwin, Zoë, 91, 186, 193
membership, 18, 20, 67, 113-14, 116, 118, 121-22, 163, 204
memory, 75, 107, 210
men's sexuality, 114
methodology, 11, 34-35, 38-39, 50
Michigan Womyn's Music Festival, 105-6, 135, 138
micro fat activism, 51, 53, 78-85, 195, 200

Venus of Willendorf, 1n2
vested interests in obesity discourse, 26, 172
Villa Magdalena K, 217

Wann, Marilyn, 12, 18, 114, 156-57, 181-82
Ward, Cathy, 207, 212
WBAI, 108-10
We Dance, 72, 132
weight loss surgery, 165-67, 171, 190, 217
West, the, 2, 18, 33, 43-44, 51, 53-54, 58, 78, 95, 131, 137, 155, 158, 160, 169, 181, 198
Westside Women's Centre, 118
white supremacy, 180-84
White, Francis Ray, 199
Whitesel, Jason, 20, 151
who benefits from research, 32
why fat feminism is obscured, 12, 21, 104, 135
Wieser, Barb, 136
witnessing, 68, 87, 200
Wogan, Terry, 98
Women's Equality Day, 125
Women's Studies, 56, 124,
Women's Therapy Centre, The, 22, 141
workshop, 41, 56, 105, 135, 148, 178, 182-84, 189, 202-4, 207-8, 210
World Health Organization (WHO), 217
Writing out of history, 18, 143

xenophobia, 131, 155

Yes!, 144

Zaps, 125, 201
Zine, 41, 48, 64-65, 71, 92, 146-47, 149, 208-10

CPSIA information can be obtained
at www.ICGtesting.com
Printed in the USA
BVHW031340240719
554234BV00008B/874/P